Manual of Screeners for Dementia

A. J. Larner

Manual of Screeners
for Dementia

Pragmatic Test Accuracy Studies

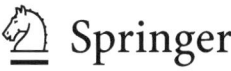 Springer

A. J. Larner
Cognitive Function Clinic
Walton Centre for Neurology
and Neurosurgery
Liverpool, UK

ISBN 978-3-030-41635-5   ISBN 978-3-030-41636-2   (eBook)
https://doi.org/10.1007/978-3-030-41636-2

This Springer imprint is published by the registered company Springer Nature Switzerland AG
The registered company address is: Gewerbestrasse 11, 6330 Cham, Switzerland

To L F

Pragmatism—is that all you have to offer?
[Tom Stoppard, Rosenkrantz and Guilden-
stern are dead]

It starts with Einstein. He shows that meas-
urement ... is not an impersonal event that
occurs with universal impartiality. It's a hu-
man act, carried out from a specific point of
view in time and space, from the one particu-
lar viewpoint of a possible observer.
[Michael Frayn, Copenhagen]

Preface

This book emerges from a conjunction of interests first partially addressed in previous volumes. Just as *Diagnostic Test Accuracy Studies in Dementia* [3, 7], a general account of the theory and practice of diagnostic test accuracy studies (DTAS), developed from Chap. 2 of *Dementia in Clinical Practice: a neurological perspective* 2nd edition [2], so the current volume is a development of Chaps. 3–6 of *Dementia in Clinical Practice: a neurological perspective* 3rd edition [5]. Specifically, it aims to highlight experience in undertaking pragmatic DTAS of screening instruments relevant to clinical practice in a dedicated cognitive disorders clinic (some of which have been included in systematic reviews, meta-analyses, and national dementia guidelines). The fact that a previous volume on cognitive screening instruments [4] achieved more than 15000 chapter downloads in less than 18 months from publication suggests an ongoing interest in and use for such tests. These constitute one aspect of a broader interest in the diagnosis of dementia and cognitive impairment [8].

To facilitate comprehension and assimilation, data are summarised in a (hopefully) easily accessible, succinct and user-friendly way by means of a structured tabular format, which should also permit ease of comparison between tests. The pragmatic study design ensures high external validity and generalisability of these test results.

The metrological tables provide an opportunity not only to document established metrics of test discrimination, such as sensitivity and specificity, predictive values and likelihood ratios, but also to explore the potentialities of some novel empirically derived unitary metrics which have been recently defined and which have not featured in previous original or summative presentations of these studies. These are the following:

- the "likelihood to diagnose or misdiagnose" (LDM; [6, 9–11, 13–15]);
- the "summary utility index" (SUI) and its reciprocal, the "number needed for screening utility" (NNSU; [10, 11]).

These metrics are easy to calculate and, I suggest, may have heuristic value. Other infrequently used "number needed" metrics (to diagnose, to predict, to misdiagnose) are also covered as these may have more intuitive appeal for clinicians, as more indicative of clinical relevance to the individual patient, than measures such as sensitivity and specificity and likelihood ratios.

An introductory chapter says more about these new metrics as they may be unfamiliar to many clinicians. The text then progresses to chapters on specific screeners which may be used in the assessment of suspected dementia and cognitive impairment, including: single-item cognitive screening questions; neurological signs; cognitive screening instruments of various lengths which may be administered to either patients or to informants; screeners for depression, functional impairment and sleep disorders; and combination and conversion of screeners. A consideration of existing and novel unitary metrics concludes the volume.

The data presented should allow clinicians to make decisions on whether these screeners are fit for purpose in their specific practice settings, being based on pragmatic diagnostic test accuracy studies. These studies were largely defined by the nature of the material encountered in a career dominated by clinical service, rather than research, issues. All were performed in accordance with STARD [1] or STARDdem [12] guidelines. All errors or misconceptions which remain in this book are entirely my own work.

Liverpool, UK   A. J. Larner, M.D. Ph.D.
a.larner@thewaltoncentre.nhs.uk

References

1. Bossuyt PM, Reitsma JB, Bruns DE, et al. The STARD statement for reporting studies of diagnostic accuracy: explanation and elaboration. Clin Chem. 2003;49:7–18.
2. Larner AJ. Dementia in clinical practice: a neurological perspective. Pragmatic studies in the Cognitive Function Clinic. 2nd ed. London: Springer;2014.
3. Larner AJ. Diagnostic test accuracy studies in dementia: a pragmatic approach. London: Springer;2015.
4. Larner AJ (ed). Cognitive screening instruments. A practical approach. 2nd ed. London: Springer;2017.
5. Larner AJ. Dementia in clinical practice: a neurological perspective. Pragmatic studies in the Cognitive Function Clinic. 3rd ed. London: Springer;2018a.
6. Larner AJ. Number needed to diagnose, predict, or misdiagnose: useful metrics for non-canonical signs of cognitive status? Dement Geriatr Cogn Dis Extra. 2018b;8:321–7.
7. Larner AJ. Diagnostic test accuracy studies in dementia. A pragmatic approach. 2nd ed. London: Springer;2019a.
8. Larner AJ (ed). Diagnosis of dementia and cognitive impairment. Basel: MDPI;2019b.
9. Larner AJ. Evaluating cognitive screening instruments with the "likelihood to be diagnosed or misdiagnosed" measure. Int J Clin Pract. 2019c;73:e13265.
10. Larner AJ. MACE for diagnosis of dementia and MCI: examining cut-offs and predictive values. Diagnostics (Basel). 2019d;9:E51.
11. Larner AJ. New unitary metrics for dementia test accuracy studies. Prog Neurol Psychiatry. 2019e;23(3):21–5.
12. Noel-Storr AH, McCleery JM, Richard E, et al. Reporting standards for studies of diagnostic test accuracy in dementia: the STARDdem Initiative. Neurology. 2014;83:364–73.

13. Williamson JC, Larner AJ. "Likelihood to be diagnosed or misdiagnosed": application to meta-analytic data for cognitive screening instruments. Neurodegener Dis Manag. 2019;9:91–5.
14. Ziso B, Larner AJ. AD8: Likelihood to diagnose or misdiagnose. J Neurol Neurosurg Psychiatry. 2019a;90:A20 (https://jnnp.bmj.com/content/90/12/A20.1).
15. Ziso B, Larner AJ. Codex (cognitive disorders examination) decision tree modified for the detection of dementia and MCI. Diagnostics (Basel). 2019b;9:E58.

Contents

Chapter 1
Introduction

1.1 Screening for Dementia

Screening for dementia and cognitive impairment may have different meanings in different contexts.

At one extreme it may refer to screening of whole populations in specific communities or areas. Epidemiological studies suggest that such populations have a low prevalence (or prior probability) of dementia and cognitive impairment. The value of screening in these situations, following the principles outlined by the World Health Organisation (WHO) screening criteria [52], is doubtful since many of the criteria are not fulfilled for dementia. For example, at time of writing no currently available pharmacotherapy for Alzheimer's disease has been shown to be more beneficial when applied at the presymptomatic/preclinical stages compared to the later symptomatic stages. Furthermore, it is not clear whether healthcare systems have sufficient capacity and policies to test for dementia and deal with the consequences, nor that the cost of case finding, including diagnosis and treatment, would be economically balanced in relation to possible expenditure on medical care as a whole [23]. Targeting at-risk groups within populations (e.g. elderly, diabetics, carriers of the apolipoprotein E epsilon 4 allele) might increase prior probability, but unfulfilled screening criteria still apply.

At the other extreme to population-based studies is the screening for dementia and cognitive impairment which takes place in dedicated memory or cognitive disorders clinics. Here the prior probability for cognitive impairment is much higher. Practically all attending individuals will have been referred with at minimum subjective memory complaints, which are recognised to increase the risk of the subsequent development of cognitive impairment [40]. The clinical encounter within these clinics, based on the clinical and informant history and physical examination, may be deemed a screening process. This is usually supplemented by the administration of dedicated cognitive screening instruments

© Springer Nature Switzerland AG 2020
A. J. Larner, *Manual of Screeners for Dementia*,
https://doi.org/10.1007/978-3-030-41636-2_1

(CSIs) or screeners. Many CSIs have been described [22, 24]. As their name implies, CSIs are not diagnostic tests but aim to facilitate identification of disease (i.e. the post-test probability is higher than prior or pre-test probability; the latter term is now used throughout, on the assumption that having reached a dedicated clinic some form of screening test, such as those described in this book, will be applied). Another approach might be to use screening instruments which attempt to exclude important differential diagnoses such as depression, or the functional cognitive disorders which are increasingly noted in memory clinics [25, 33]. Increased post-test probability will allow the appropriate targeting of more sophisticated (and expensive) investigations for diagnosis and hence treatment.

Of course, it should be realised that screening strategies for dementia and cognitive impairment using investigations other than CSIs exist or may be conceived. One might use genetic epidemiology to construct "polygenic hazard scores" for the development of AD [11, 35]. This approach is illustrative of the emerging focus on construction of risk prediction models or "bioprediction" of brain disorder. Constructing a probability function, a probabilistic model based on present and future risks of harm, might be used to address individual risk of developing Alzheimer's disease. "Risk banding", based on the shape of the probability function, is a strategy which might be used to determine the necessity or otherwise for response/intervention [2].

The purpose of this book is to examine the utility of CSIs using various metrics derived from pragmatic test accuracy studies (Sect. 1.2).

1.2   Pragmatic Test Accuracy Studies

The methodology of test accuracy studies is well established [16, 28]. Sackett and Haynes [50] described an "architecture of diagnostic research" which proposed four relevant types or phases, of which phase III asks whether test results distinguish those with and without the target disorder among those in whom it is clinically sensible to suspect the target disorder. This seems to me to describe the day-to-day clinical situation encountered in cognitive disorders clinics, prompting my use of the descriptors "pragmatic diagnostic test accuracy studies" [20] or "pragmatic screening test accuracy studies" [28, p. 8–10]. The latter type of study has been pursued in the author's clinic over the past 15 years.

Unlike phase I/II studies [50], also known as experimental or proof-of-concept studies, pragmatic or observational studies have a number of advantages [28, p. 172–5]. There is no control group, as befits clinical practice where no controls attend for consultation. This approach also minimises restrictive inclusion/exclusion criteria, making study recruitment easier with more generalizable study results because of the high external validity. Such studies could potentially be undertaken in any clinic, and not restricted to research settings. Pragmatic test accuracy studies are more stringent, more exacting, in their evaluation of CSIs than experimental or proof-of-concept studies, with consequently less risk of over-inflating study outcomes when using a healthy control group.

The presentation of the study data is critical for accurate dissemination of the study findings. In this volume, a standardized tabulation of data is presented for each screener, covering demographic and measurement parameters (Fig. 1.1). Of course, these data are not exhaustive, but in balancing comprehensiveness with the risk of data overload some of the available parameters have been omitted, including diagnostic odds ratio, area under the receiver operating characteristic curve, net reclassification improvement, and effect sizes, many of which have their own shortcomings and all of which have been discussed elsewhere [26, 28] (see also Sect. 14.2).

1.3   Data Presentation

1.3.1   Standard Metrics

Many of the test metrics which are included will be very familiar and therefore require little discussion [28, 47]. All these metrics may be derived from the 2×2 contingency table (or confusion matrix/table) which cross-classifies the reference standard or criterion diagnosis ("true status") with the test outcome (Fig. 1.2). The latter is dichotomised according to a chosen threshold, cut-off or cut-point. The cut-off is usually established (and fixed) by the index study of the particular test in question, and there are various methods which may be used to do this.

Sensitivity (Sens) and specificity (Spec), the correct identification of true positives and true negatives (i.e. true positive rate, TPR, and true negative rate, TNR, respectively), are recommended as keywords of papers reporting diagnostic test accuracy studies in both the STAndards for the Reporting of Diagnostic accuracy studies (STARD; [5]) and STARDdem [42] guidelines. There is a trade-off between these parameters and their complements, false negative rate (FNR = 1 − TPR) and false positive rate (FPR = 1 − TNR). A test with high sensitivity has few false negatives, and hence a negative test is likely to be a true negative and hence rules out the diagnosis (so called "SnNout" rule). Conversely, a test with low sensitivity has many false negatives, and hence misses cases. A test with high specificity has few false positives, and hence a positive test is likely to be a true positive and hence rules in the diagnosis (so called "SpPin" rule). Conversely, a test with low specificity has many false positives, and hence misidentifies non cases as cases.

Positive and negative predictive values (PPV, NPV) are often cited measures of probability, denoting respectively the proportion of subjects with a positive test who have disease, and of subjects with a negative test who do not have the disease.

Likelihood ratios (LR+, LR−) combine information about sensitivity and specificity [45] to give, respectively, the odds of a positive test result in an affected individual relative to an unaffected, and the odds of a negative test result in an

1. Demographics:

N	The total number of patients in the study cohort who were administered both the index test and independently the reference standard
P = Prevalence rate	P = The probability of a patient having the diagnosis of interest: P = (True positives + False negatives)/Total number tested Depending on the study, P may be the diagnosis of dementia, or mild cognitive impairment, or any cognitive impairment (dementia + MCI), or no cognitive impairment P = prior or pre-test probability. If required, the pre-test odds may be calculated from this, as P/(1 − P) or P/ P'
Q = Level of the test	Q = The probability of a patient having a positive test in the population studied, the "positive sign rate": Q = (True positives + False positives)/Total number tested

2. Paired measures of discrimination:

Sensitivity (Sens) Specificity (Spec)	Sens = True positives/(True positives + False negatives) Spec = True negatives/(False positives + True negatives) Range 0 to 1, higher better
Positive predictive value (PPV) Negative predictive value (NPV)	PPV = True positives/(True positives + False positives) This value is equal to the post-test probability NPV = True negatives/(False negatives + True negatives) Range 0 to 1, higher better
Positive likelihood ratio (LR+) Negative likelihood ratio (LR−)	LR+ = Sens/(1 − Spec), = how many times more likely positive findings are in people with compared to without the condition Range 1 to ∞, higher better If required, the post-test odds may be calculated from LR+ x pre-test odds LR− = (1 − Sens)/Spec, = how many times less likely negative findings are in people with compared to without the condition Range 0 to 1, lower better
Positive clinical utility index (CUI+) Negative clinical utility index (CUI−)	CUI+ = Sens × PPV CUI− = Spec × NPV Range 0 to 1, higher better

Fig. 1.1 Standard metrological tables used throughout this book, summarising pragmatic test accuracy studies of cognitive screeners (see also Fig. 1.2)

3. Unitary measures of discrimination:

Accuracy (Acc)	Acc = (True positives + True negatives)/Total number tested Range 0 to 1, higher better This value is equal to the posterior probability
Youden index (Y)	Y = (Sens + Spec) − 1 Range −1 to 1, higher better
Predictive summary index (PSI, or Ψ)	PSI = (PPV + NPV) − 1 Range −1 to 1, higher better
Summary utility index (SUI)	SUI = (CUI+ + CUI−) See Sect. 1.3.5 and Table 1.3

4. Numbers needed:

To diagnose (NND)	NND = 1/Y Lower value better See Sect. 1.3.3
To predict (NNP)	NNP = 1/PSI Lower value better See Sect. 1.3.3
To misdiagnose (NNM)	NNM = 1/(1 − Acc) or 1/Inaccuracy Higher value better See Sect. 1.3.3
Likelihood to be diagnosed or misdiagnosed (LDM)	LDM = NNM/NND or NNM/NNP Higher value better See Sect. 1.3.4
For screening utility (NNSU)	NNSU = 1/SUI See Sect. 1.3.5 and Table 1.4

Fig. 1.1 (continued)

affected individual relative to an unaffected. A likelihood ratio >1 indicates that the test result is associated with the presence of disease; a likelihood ratio <1 indicates that the test result is associated with the absence of disease [10]. Likelihood ratios were used for the evidence statements in the Dementia Guideline issued by the United Kingdom National Institute for Health and Care Excellence [41].

Clinical utility indexes (CUI+, CUI−) respectively comprise the product of Sens and PPV, used as a measure of ruling in a diagnosis, and the product of Spec and NPV, a measure of ruling out a diagnosis [39]. CUIs may be less familiar than the aforementioned paired measures, although have been used in the evaluation of some CSIs [15] and may be included amongst standard summary measures of discrimination [3], as has been the case in studies performed in the author's clinic [28, p. 125, 126].

Some of these metrics have qualitative classifications as well as numerical values; specifically, of those used here, likelihood ratios [14] (see Table 1.1) and

		True Status	
		Condition present	**Condition absent**
Test Outcome	**Positive**	True positive [TP]	False positive [FP]
	Negative	False negative [FN]	True negative [TN]

Marginal value probabilities:

$$
\begin{aligned}
P &= (TP + FN)/N \\
(1 - P) = P' &= (FP + TN)/N \\
Q &= (TP + FP)/N \\
(1 - Q) = Q' &= (FN + TN)/N
\end{aligned}
$$

Paired measures:

$$
\begin{aligned}
\text{Sens (TPR)} &= TP/(TP + FN) \\
\text{Spec (TNR)} &= TN/(FP + TN) \\[1em]
FPR &= (1 - TNR) = FP/(FP + TN) \\
FNR &= (1 - TPR) = FN/(TP + FN) \\[1em]
PPV &= TP/(TP + FP) \\
NPV &= TN/(FN + TN) \\[1em]
LR+ &= [TP/(TP + FN)]/[FP/(FP + TN)] \\
LR- &= [FN/(TP + FN)]/[TN/(FP + TN)] \\[1em]
CUI+ &= \text{Sens} \times PPV \\
CUI- &= \text{Spec} \times NPV
\end{aligned}
$$

Fig. 1.2 Diagnostic test accuracy study 2×2 table with marginal value probabilities and paired measures

Table 1.1 Classification of LRs (after Jaeschke et al. [14])

LR value	Qualitative classification: change in probability of disease	Previously used nomenclature [26]
$LR- \leq 0.1$	Very large decrease	Large
$0.1 < LR- \leq 0.2$	Large decrease	Moderate
$0.2 < LR- \leq 0.5$	Moderate decrease	Small
$0.5 < LR- \leq 1.0$	Slight decrease	Unimportant
$1.0 < LR+ < 2.0$	Slight increase	Unimportant
$2.0 \leq LR+ < 5.0$	Moderate increase	Small
$5.0 \leq LR+ < 10.0$	Large increase	Moderate
$LR+ \geq 10.0$	Very large increase	Large

Table 1.2   Classification of CUIs (after Mitchell [39])

	Excellent	Good	Adequate	Poor	Very poor
CUI+, CUI−	≥0.81	≥0.64	≥0.49	≥0.36	<0.36

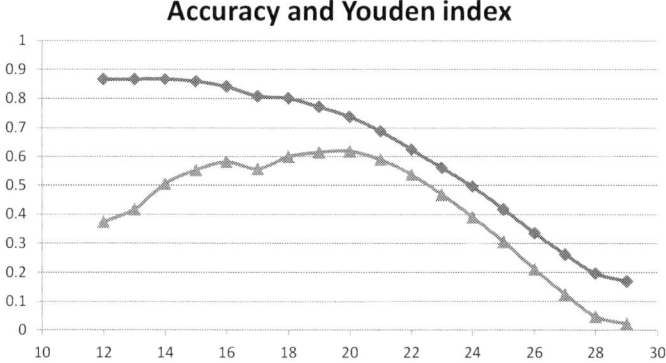

Fig. 1.3 Plot of Accuracy (upper line) and of Youden index (lower line) against MACE cut-off (x-axis; unpublished data from Larner [29]: note different maxima, ≤14/30 and ≤20/30 respectively)

clinical utility indexes [39] (see Table 1.2). The qualitative classifications of these test results are included in each of the metrological tables.

There are a number of global or unitary measures of test accuracy, of which accuracy or correct classification accuracy (Acc) is probably the most familiar. The Youden index ($Y = Sens + Spec - 1$) is also sometimes used (Sect. 1.3.3).

It is obvious that the method chosen to establish the test cut-off value will influence all the metrics which are derived from the 2×2 table. For example, using maximal test accuracy or maximal test Youden index will produce different cut-offs [21, 43]; the optima of other unitary measures may also be used to determine cut-offs [34]. As an example, using data from a test accuracy study of the Mini-Addenbrooke's Cognitive Examination (MACE; [29]), values of accuracy and Youden index have been plotted against differing test cut-offs to demonstrate the different maxima obtained using the two methods (Fig. 1.3; maximal accuracy at MACE cut-off ≤14/30, maximal Youden index at MACE cut-off ≤20/30).

The possibility of error in the reference standard or criterion diagnosis (i.e. misdiagnosis) can also affect test metrics. Although reference diagnoses are generally based on widely accepted diagnostic criteria, errors may nevertheless occur, particularly when patient assessment is cross-sectional as opposed to longitudinal, the latter providing the opportunity for delayed verification of diagnoses, perhaps even at post mortem [12]. Misdiagnosis may occur for various reasons, but over-reliance on reports of structural brain imaging may be a particular theme [9, 18, 48]. There are some test metrics which specifically address the possibility of misdiagnosis (Sects. 1.3.3 and 1.3.4).

Other test measures which are used in the summary data tables may be less familiar than those mentioned hitherto, and hence are described in more detail below (Sects. 1.3.3, 1.3.4, and 1.3.5).

1.3.2   Prevalence (P) and Level (Q)

Study setting and type determines disease frequency or prevalence rate (P). Prevalence is an indication of disease burden in a given population. The pre-test probability of the target disease is given by P. The pre-test probability of the absence of disease is given by $(1 - P)$ or P'. P is influenced by the chosen study population, based on location (community, primary, secondary care) and study type (experimental or observational).

Test performance may differ in different settings, related in part to P. Rescaling of test metrics to take P into account may be necessary. Provision of figures for sensitivity and specificity for each pragmatic study discussed in subsequent chapters will permit easy calculation of predictive values at different chosen levels of disease prevalence, using standard equations:

$$PPV = Sens \times P/(Sens \times P) + [(1 - Spec) \times P'] \qquad (1.1)$$

$$NPV = Spec \times P'/[Spec \times P'] + [(1 - Sens) \times P] \qquad (1.2)$$

Likewise for correct classification accuracy (Acc), the weighted average of sensitivity and specificity with weights equal to sample prevalence (P):

$$Acc = Sens \times P + Spec \times P' \qquad (1.3)$$

Such calculations for predictive values have been reported for some screening instruments at prevalence rates of 5, 10, 20, and 40%, including the Addenbrooke's Cognitive Examination (ACE), its revised version (ACE-R), and MACE [29]. This adjustment also permits calculation of other parameters related to prevalence, including predictive summary index and its reciprocal (Sect. 1.3.3), clinical utility indexes, one formulation of the likelihood to be diagnosed or misdiagnosed metric (Sect. 1.3.4), and the summary utility index and its reciprocal (Sect. 1.3.5).

Kraemer [17] developed a metric, Q, the level of a test, also known as the "positive sign rate". The probability of a positive test in the patient population is Q. The probability of a negative test in the patient population ("negative sign rate") is $1 - Q$ or Q'. From these values of Q and Q', quality sensitivity and specificity (QSN, QSP) values may be calculated which give the increment in each parameter beyond the level, such that:

$$QSN = (Sens - Q)/Q'$$
$$QSP = (Spec - Q')/Q$$

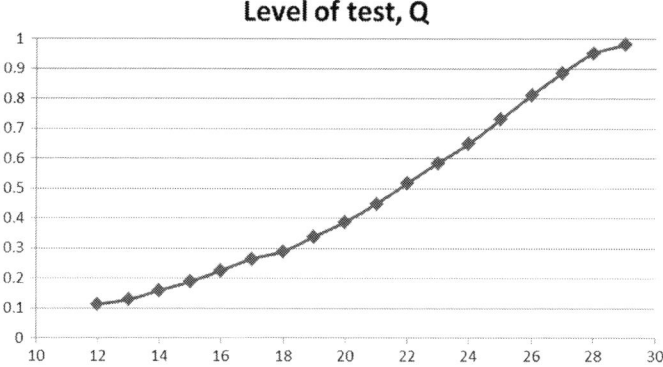

Fig. 1.4 Plot of level of test, Q, against MACE cut-off (x-axis; unpublished data from Larner [29])

It has been suggested that these calibrated, rescaled, or standardized indices of test parameters are more comparable across different samples [30, 36].

In pragmatic studies the level of the test, Q, is determined by the choice of test cut-off (Fig. 1.4). The more sensitive the test, the more positives, both true and false, are identified.

1.3.3 "Number Needed" (NN) Metrics

"Number needed to" metrics were developed to summarise impact in a manner more intuitive to clinicians and patients than the traditional measures of discrimination such as sensitivity and specificity.

In the context of therapeutics, Cook and Sackett [8] developed the "number needed to treat" (NNT), which was later followed by the "number needed to harm" (NNH; [54]). Both NNT and NNH are established concepts for most clinicians. Other adaptations have also been made, such as the "number needed to see" for a specific occurrence to be encountered in clinical practice (NNS; [19]). "Number needed to screen" (also abbreviated as NNS) metrics have been defined, both for purposes of public health epidemiology (as the number of people that need to be screened for a given duration to prevent one death or adverse event; [49]) or diagnostic test accuracy (number of patients who need to be screened in order for one additional correct identification beyond those misidentified; [38]; see Sect. 1.3.5 for further discussion).

Youden [53] developed an index, Y, of the sum of the two fractions showing proportions correctly diagnosed in diseased and non-diseased groups diminished by unity:

$$Y = (Sens + Spec) - 1 \qquad (1.4)$$

Although Y may range from -1 to 1, most values would be expected to fall within the range 0 (no diagnostic value) to 1 (no false positives or false negatives), with negative values occurring only if the test were misleading, i.e. the test result was negatively associated with the true diagnosis.

The reciprocal or multiplicative inverse of the Youden index, $1/Y$, has been defined by Linn and Grunau [37] as the "number needed to diagnose" (NND), that is the number of patients who need to be examined in order to detect correctly one person with the disease of interest in a study population of persons with and without the known disease:

$$NND = 1/Y \qquad (1.5)$$

For diagnostic tests, low values of NND will be desirable. Assuming no negative values for Y, NND may range from infinity ($Y = 0$, no diagnostic value) to 1 ($Y = 1$). As the value of Y approaches 0, NND values become inflated, as is the case for any multiplicative inverse, an observation which has prompted the opinion that NND is not a clinically meaningful number [38].

NND is insensitive to variation in disease prevalence, since it depends entirely on sensitivity and specificity. To address this deficiency, Linn and Grunau [37] suggested further new statistics. The predictive summary index (PSI or Ψ) is a unitary measure of test performance defined as:

$$PSI = (PPV + NPV) - 1 \qquad (1.6)$$

which reflects total net gain in certainty (Fig. 1.1). Like Y, PSI may range from -1 to 1, although negative values are not anticipated. The multiplicative inverse of PSI ($1/PSI$ or $1/\Psi$) was termed the "number needed to predict" (NNP), interpreted as the number of patients who need to be examined in the patient population in order to predict correctly diagnosis of one person:

$$NNP = 1/PSI \qquad (1.7)$$

NNP is dependent on prevalence and may therefore be deemed a better descriptor of diagnostic tests in patient populations with different prevalence of disease. For diagnostic tests, low values of NNP will be desirable. Assuming no negative values for PSI, NNP may range from infinity (PSI$=0$, no diagnostic value) to 1 (PSI$=1$).

Habibzadeh and Yadollahie [13] proposed another index, the "number needed to misdiagnose" (NNM), as a measure of diagnostic test effectiveness, defined as the inverse of $(1 - Acc)$ or Inaccuracy (Fig. 1.1):

$$NNM = 1/Inacc = 1/(1 - Acc) \qquad (1.8)$$

Inaccuracy (Inacc) may range from 0 (all true positives and true negatives identified, i.e. accuracy $= 1$) to 1 (no diagnostic value). NNM is the number of patients who need to be tested in order for one to be misdiagnosed by the test. For diagnostic tests, high values of NNM will be desirable. NNM may range from infinity (Inacc $= 0$, perfect test) to 1 (Inacc $= 1$, no diagnostic value).

Because "number needed" metrics refer to patients, it is obvious that only positive integer values are clinically meaningful. Hence, their absolute ("raw") values should be rounded to the next highest integer value for purposes of clinical communication (e.g. as in Larner [29], Tables 3 and 6). Whilst it is possible to define the probability of non-events mathematically (e.g. $(1 - P)$ or P'), this cannot be extended to non-persons!

A further "number needed" metric has also been developed, based on clinical utility indexes (see Sect. 1.3.5).

1.3.4   Likelihood to be Diagnosed or Misdiagnosed (LDM)

Using the "number needed" metrics developed to describe therapeutic studies (i.e. NNT, NNH), Citrome and Ketter [6] described a "likelihood to be helped or harmed" (LHH) metric, calculated as the ratio of the number needed to harm to the number needed to treat (NNH/NNT). Since NNH is desirably as large as possible (ideally infinite), and NNT is desirably as small as possible (ideally 1), LHH values are ideally as large as possible. LHH is reported to help "both clinician and patient evaluate potential risk-benefit trade-offs with treatment" [1].

An analogous, novel, metric has been derived for test accuracy studies, and called the "likelihood to be diagnosed or misdiagnosed" (LDM; [27, 29, 31, 32]). This is calculated as the ratio of NNM to either NND or NNP:

$$LDM = NNM/NND$$
$$= [1/(1 - Acc)]/1/Y \qquad (1.9)$$

or

$$LDM = NNM/NNP$$
$$= [1/(1 - Acc)]/1/PSI \qquad (1.10)$$

LDM helps both clinician and patient evaluate potential risk-benefit trade-offs with particular diagnostic tests. Since for diagnostic tests low values of NND and NNP and high values of NNM are desirable, higher values of LDM (>1) would suggest a test more likely to favour diagnosis over misdiagnosis, whereas lower values of LDM (<1) favour misdiagnosis over diagnosis.

LDM has been calculated for some non-canonical neurological signs ("attended alone" sign and its converse, the "attended with" sign; the head turning sign, the applause sign, and *la maladie du petit papier*) and cognitive screening instruments (MMSE, MoCA, MACE, 6CIT, AD8, Codex; [27, 29, 31, 32, 55, 56]). It may be desirable to extend analysis using this metric to other screening and diagnostic tests, and to meta-analytic data [51, 55].

1.3.5   Summary Utility Index (SUI) and its Reciprocal (NNSU)

Mitchell [39] proposed a "clinical utility index" (CUI), defined as $CUI+ = Sens \times PPV$ (also called the "screening marker index" by Ostergaard et al. [44]), and $CUI- = Spec \times NPV$ (Sect. 1.3.1). These paired indices were developed in order to take into account both occurrence and discrimination, and may be used as markers respectively to rule in and rule out diagnosis [39]. Clinical utility indexes have been used extensively in previous pragmatic diagnostic test accuracy studies undertaken in this clinic [26].

As single, global, or unitary indices may be helpful in defining utility of diagnostic tests, such as the Youden index (Y; [53]) and the predictive summary index (PSI; 37), the possibility of combining CUIs in a metric with heuristic value for text accuracy studies was considered [32] and different methods for its construction explored.

One way to define a "summary utility index" (SUI) is by simple analogy with Y and PSI:

$$\text{Method 1: SUI} = (CUI+ \; + \; CUI-) - 1$$

This proposes SUI as the sum of the two fractions showing proportions for which the test has clinical utility for diseased and non-diseased groups diminished by unity. SUI would thus, like Y and PSI, range from 1 to -1, and would desirably be as close to 1 as possible. More precisely, such SUI values could be qualitatively classified, using the classification of CUIs suggested by Mitchell [39] (see Table 1.2), as shown in Table 1.3, Method 1.

As previously mentioned, "number needed" metrics may be derived from Y and PSI, respectively the number needed to diagnose (NND) and number needed to predict (NNP; Sect. 1.3.3). By analogy, it is possible to propose a "number needed for screening utility" (NNSU) metric, defined as the reciprocal or multiplicative inverse of SUI:

$$NNSU \; = 1/SUI$$

However, this formulation proved problematic in practice because, pragmatically, many SUI values were negative (unlike the situation anticipated with Y and PSI; see Sect. 1.3.3). Hence negative and clinically meaningless values for NNSU were obtained, a reflection of the fact that multiplicative inverse functions are discontinuous and asymptotic with the y axis.

Table 1.3 Classification of SUI (after Larner [32])

	Excellent	Good	Adequate	Poor	Very poor
Method 1: (CUI+ + CUI−) − 1	≥0.62	≥0.28	≥−0.06	≥−0.28	<−0.28
Method 2: (CUI+ + CUI−)	≥1.62	≥1.28	≥0.98	≥0.72	<0.72

Analogous reasoning tends to emphasise similarities whilst minimising or ignoring differences. For example, Y is derived as the difference between the true positive rate (TPR, i.e. sensitivity) and the false positive rate (FPR), the complement or negation of specificity (i.e. FPR = 1 − specificity), hence:

$$Y = TPR − FPR$$
$$= Sens − (1 − Spec)$$
$$= (Sens + Spec) − 1 \qquad (1.4)$$

Likewise, for PSI, which is the difference between the positive predictive value and the false reassurance rate (FRR; also known as false omission rate), the complement or negation of negative predictive value (i.e. FRR = 1 − NPV), hence:

$$PSI = PPV − FRR$$
$$= PPV − (1 − NPV)$$
$$= (PPV + NPV) − 1 \qquad (1.6)$$

CUI+ and CUI− are not rates like TPR, FPR, PPV, and FRR, so such derivations do not apply.

For heuristics, it may thus be better to acknowledge the shortcomings of SUI Method 1 and, particularly, of NNSU derived therefrom, computed as analogues of Y and NND and PSI and NNP, and instead attempt a different formulation.

Most easily this might be done by simple addition of CUI+ and CUI−, a method analogous to the sum of sensitivity and specificity which has been termed "gain in certainty" [7] or overall correct classification rate [46]. Hence:

$$\text{Method 2}: \ SUI = (CUI+ + CUI−) \qquad (1.11)$$

In this case SUI may range from 0 to 2, and would desirably be as close to 2 as possible. It follows that SUIs would then be classified as in Table 1.3, Method 2. This is the calculation method and qualitative classification of SUI which is included in each metrological table in this book.

Negative values of SUI are now not possible, rather than simply unanticipated, as is the case for Y and PSI. Hence:

$$NNSU = 1/SUI$$
$$= 1/(CUI+ + CUI−) \qquad (1.12)$$

such that all NNSU values are now positive, with anticipated range of ∞ (SUI = 0, no screening value) to 0.5 (SUI = 2, perfect screening utility), with low values of NNSU desirable.

Following the qualitative classification of SUI (Table 1.3, Method 2), it is also possible to classify NNSU values qualitatively (Table 1.4). More generally NNSU values may be dichotomised, as <1 being acceptable or desirable, >1 not so ("inadequate"). Hence, as for other "number needed" metrics (Sect. 1.3.1), NNSU calculated by this method may be of intuitive value for clinicians and patients.

SUI and NNSU have been calculated for some non-canonical neurological signs ("attended alone" sign and its converse, the "attended with" sign; the head turning sign, the applause sign, and *la maladie du petit papier*) and cognitive screening instruments (MMSE, MoCA, MACE, 6CIT, AD8) and were easy to classify [32].

The general term "summary utility index" (SUI) might be further qualified according to context as either a "summary screening utility index" (SSUI) or "summary diagnostic utility index" (SDUI) dependent upon whether screening or diagnostic tests are being examined. Following Connell and Koepsell [7], SUI might be characterised as either the "gain in screening utility" or "gain in diagnostic utility" of a test, and following Perkins and Schisterman [46] as the "overall correct screening rate".

It is instructive to compare NNSU with the "number needed to screen" (NNS) metric defined by Mitchell [38]. The latter is derived from an identification index (II), where:

$$II = Acc - (Inacc)$$
$$= Acc - (1 - Acc)$$
$$= 2 \times Acc - 1$$

From which:

$$NNS = 1/II$$
$$= 1/Acc - (Inacc)$$
$$= 1/Acc - (1 - Acc)$$
$$= 1/2 \times Acc - 1$$

For this argument, the shortcoming of Acc (Fig. 1.1) as a measure which treats false positives and false negatives as equally undesirable is accepted, even though this is often not necessarily the case in clinical practice [4]. As for Y and PSI (Sect. 1.3.3), II may range from -1 to 1. However, whereas negative values are not anticipated with Y and PSI, any value of Acc <0.5 (i.e. Inacc >0.5) will result in a negative II, and hence a negative NNS. As previously mentioned, only positive integer values are clinically meaningful for "number needed" metrics (NND, NNP, and NNM; Sect. 1.3.3) since these refer to patients, so negative NNS values are clinically meaningless.

The fact that NNSU cannot be <0, since by definition SUI cannot be <0, avoids this problem encountered with NNS, although not the inevitable inflation of NNSU at low values of SUI. A comparison of NNS and NNSU at a range of

Table 1.4 Classification of NNSU (after Larner [32])

	Excellent	Good	Adequate
Method 2: NNSU = 1/SUI = 1/(CUI+ +CUI−)	$0.5 \leq NNSU \leq 0.62$	$0.62 < NNSU \leq 0.78$	$0.78 < NNSU \leq 1.02$

test cut-offs was examined in a study of the Mini-Addenbrooke's Cognitive Examination, illustrating this point and suggesting the advantage of using NNSU over NNS [29] (Tables 3 and 6). Moreover, NNS lacks a qualitative classification as per NNSU (Table 1.4).

References

1. Andrade C. Likelihood of being helped or harmed as a measure of clinical outcomes in psychopharmacology. J Clin Psychiatry. 2017;78:e73–5.
2. Baum ML. The neuroethics of biomarkers. What the development of bioprediction means for moral responsibility, justice, and the nature of mental disorder. Oxford: Oxford University Press; 2016.
3. Bolboaca SD. Medical diagnostic tests: a review of test anatomy, phases, and statistical treatment of data. Comput Math Methods Med. 2019;2019:1891569.
4. Bossuyt PMM. Clinical validity: defining biomarker performance. Scand J Clin Lab Invest. 2010;70 Suppl 242:46–52.
5. Bossuyt PM, Reitsma JB, Bruns DE, et al. The STARD statement for reporting studies of diagnostic accuracy: explanation and elaboration. Clin Chem. 2003;49:7–18.
6. Citrome L, Ketter TA. When does a difference make a difference? Interpretation of number needed to treat, number needed to harm, and likelihood to be helped or harmed. Int J Clin Pract. 2013;67:407–11.
7. Connell FA, Koepsell TD. Measures of gain in certainty from a diagnostic test. Am J Epidemiol. 1985;121:744–53.
8. Cook RJ, Sackett DL. The number needed to treat: a clinically useful measure of treatment effect. BMJ. 1995;310:452–4.
9. Davies M, Larner AJ. Clinical misdiagnosis of Alzheimer's disease: getting it wrong again. Eur J Neurol. 2009;16 Suppl 3:351 (abstract 2036).
10. Deeks JJ, Altman DG. Diagnostic tests 4: likelihood ratios. BMJ. 2004;329:168–9.
11. Desikan RS, Fan CC, Wang Y, et al. Genetic assessment of age-associated Alzheimer disease risk: development and validation of a polygenic hazard score. PLoS Med. 2017;14(3):e1002258.
12. Du Plessis DG, Larner AJ. Phenotypic similarities causing clinical misdiagnosis of pathologically-confirmed sporadic Creutzfeldt-Jakob disease as dementia with Lewy bodies. Clin Neurol Neurosurg. 2008;110:194–7.
13. Habibzadeh F, Yadollahie M. Number needed to misdiagnose: a measure of diagnostic test effectiveness. Epidemiology. 2013;24:170.
14. Jaeschke R, Guyatt G, Sackett DL. Users' guide to the medical literature. III. How to use an article about a diagnostic test. B. What are the results and will they help me in caring for my patients? JAMA. 1994;271:703–7.
15. Johansson MM, Kvitting AS, Wressle E, Marcusson J. Clinical utility of cognistat in multiprofessional team evaluations of patients with cognitive impairment in Swedish primary care. Int J Family Med. 2014;2014:649253.
16. Knottnerus JA, editor. The evidence base of clinical diagnosis. London: BMJ Books; 2002.
17. Kraemer HC. Evaluating medical tests. Objective and quantitative guidelines. Newbery Park, California: Sage; 1992.
18. Larner AJ. Getting it wrong: the clinical misdiagnosis of Alzheimer's disease. Int J Clin Pract. 2004;58:1092–4.
19. Larner AJ. Teleneurology by internet and telephone. A study of medical self-help. London: Springer; 2011.

20. Larner AJ. Pragmatic diagnostic accuracy studies. http://bmj.com/content/345/bmj. e3999?tab=responses, 28 August 2012.
21. Larner AJ. Optimizing the cutoffs of cognitive screening instruments in pragmatic diagnostic accuracy studies: maximising accuracy or Youden index? Dement Geriatr Cogn Disord. 2015;39:167–75.
22. Larner AJ (ed.). Cognitive screening instruments. A practical approach. 2nd ed. London: Springer; 2017.
23. Larner AJ. Dementia and the health of the nation. In: Severn A, editor. Cognitive changes after surgery in clinical practice. London: Springer; 2018a. p. 1–15.
24. Larner AJ. Assessment of cognitive function. In: Severn A, editor. Cognitive changes after surgery in clinical practice. London: Springer; 2018b. p. 45–60.
25. Larner AJ. Dementia screening: a different proposal. Future Neurol. 2018c;13:177–9.
26. Larner AJ. Dementia in clinical practice: a neurological perspective. Pragmatic studies in the Cognitive Function Clinic. 3rd ed. London: Springer; 2018d.
27. Larner AJ. Number needed to diagnose, predict, or misdiagnose: useful metrics for non-canonical signs of cognitive status? Dement Geriatr Cogn Dis Extra. 2018e;8:321–7.
28. Larner AJ. Diagnostic test accuracy studies in dementia. A pragmatic approach. 2nd ed. London: Springer; 2019a.
29. Larner AJ. MACE for diagnosis of dementia and MCI: examining cut-offs and predictive values. Diagnostics (Basel). 2019b;9:E51.
30. Larner AJ. Applying Kraemer's Q (positive sign rate): some implications for diagnostic test accuracy study results. Dement Geriatr Cogn Dis Extra. 2019c:9:389–96.
31. Larner AJ. Evaluating cognitive screening instruments with the "likelihood to be diagnosed or misdiagnosed" measure. Int J Clin Pract. 2019d;73:e13265.
32. Larner AJ. New unitary metrics for dementia test accuracy studies. Prog Neurol Psychiatry. 2019e;23(3):21–5.
33. Larner AJ. Functional cognitive disorders: update on diagnostic status. Neurodegener Dis Manag. 2020a;10:in press.
34. Larner AJ. Defining "optimal" test cut-off using global test metrics: evidence from a cognitive screening instrument. 2020b;submitted.
35. Larner AJ, Bracewell RM. Predicting Alzheimer's disease: a polygenic hazard score. J R Coll Physicians Edinb. 2017;47:151–2.
36. Larrabee GJ, Barry DTR. Diagnostic classification statistics and diagnostic validity of malingering assessment. In: Larrabee GJ, editor. Assessment of malingered neuropsychological deficits. Oxford: Oxford University Press; 2007. p. 14–26.
37. Linn S, Grunau PD. New patient-oriented summary measure of net total gain in certainty for dichotomous diagnostic tests. Epidemiol Perspect Innov. 2006;3:11.
38. Mitchell AJ. Index test. In: Kattan MW, editor. Encyclopedia of medical decision making. Los Angeles: Sage; 2009. p. 613–7.
39. Mitchell AJ. Sensitivity × PPV is a recognized test called the clinical utility index (CUI+). Eur J Epidemiol. 2011;26:251–2.
40. Mitchell AJ, Beaumont H, Ferguson D, Yadegarfar M, Stubbs B. Risk of dementia and mild cognitive impairment in older people with subjective memory complaints: meta-analysis. Acta Psychiatr Scand. 2014;130:439–51.
41. National Institute for Health and Care Excellence. Dementia. Assessment, management and support for people living with dementia and their carers. NICE Guideline 97. Methods, evidence and recommendations. London: NICE; 2018.
42. Noel-Storr AH, McCleery JM, Richard E, et al. Reporting standards for studies of diagnostic test accuracy in dementia: the STARDdem Initiative. Neurology. 2014;83:364–73.
43. O'Caoimh R, Gao Y, Svendovski A, Gallagher P, Eustace J, Molloy DW. Comparing approaches to optimize cut-off scores for short cognitive screening instruments in mild cognitive impairment and dementia. J Alzheimers Dis. 2017;57:123–33.

44. Ostergaard SD, Dinesen PT, Foldager L. Quantifying the value of markers in screening pro-grammes. Eur J Epidemiol. 2010;25:151–4.
45. Perera R, Heneghan C. Making sense of diagnostic tests likelihood ratios. Evid Based Med. 2006;11:130–1.
46. Perkins NJ, Schisterman EF. The inconsistency of "optimal" cutpoints obtained using two criteria based on the receiver operating characteristic curve. Am J Epidemiol. 2006;163:670–5.
47. Quinn TJ, Takwoingi Y. Assessment of the utility of cognitive screening instruments. In: Larner AJ, editor. Cognitive screening instruments. A practical approach. 2nd ed. London: Springer; 2017. p. 15–34.
48. Randall A, Larner AJ. Primary progressive aphasia: misdiagnosis with "normal imaging". Prog Neurol Psychiatry. 2020;24:in press.
49. Rembold CM. Number needed to screen: development of a statistic for disease screening. BMJ. 1998;317:307–12.
50. Sackett DL, Haynes RB. The architecture of diagnostic research. In: Knottnerus JA, editor. The evidence base of clinical diagnosis. London: BMJ Books; 2002. p. 19–38.
51. Williamson JC, Larner AJ. "Likelihood to be diagnosed or misdiagnosed": applica-tion to meta-analytic data for cognitive screening instruments. Neurodegener Dis Manag. 2019;9:91–5.
52. Wilson JMG, Jungner G. Principles and practice of screening for disease. Public health paper no. 34. Geneva: World Health Organisation; 1968.
53. Youden WJ. Index for rating diagnostic tests. Cancer. 1950;3:32–5.
54. Zermansky A. Number needed to harm should be measured for treatments. BMJ. 1998;317:1014.
55. Ziso B, Larner AJ. AD8: Likelihood to diagnose or misdiagnose. J Neurol Neurosurg Psychiatry. 2019a;90:A20 (https://jnnp.bmj.com/content/90/12/A20.1).
56. Ziso B, Larner AJ. Codex (cognitive disorders examination) decision tree modified for the detection of dementia and MCI. Diagnostics (Basel). 2019b;9:E58.

Chapter 2
Single-Item Cognitive Screening Questions

2.1 Introduction

Single-item cognitive screening questions are an attractive proposition because of their simplicity. They are quick and easy to use, and generally acceptable to patients and informants. They provide categorical answers.

A systematic review of single screening questions for cognitive impairment in older people found 11 eligible studies (from 884 titles screened), with sensitivity range 0.26–0.96 and specificity range 0.45–1.00. The review conclusion was that informant-based single-item screening questions for cognitive impairment showed promise but there was currently insufficient evidence to support routine use [6].

It should be noted that the single-item cognitive screeners discussed here have been examined in a high prevalence secondary care setting (P for cognitive impairment of around 0.5), so calculations adjusting for the lower disease prevalence anticipated in primary care and community settings may be undertaken using standard equations (Sect. 1.3.2, Eqs. 1.1 and 1.2).

2.2 Dementia CQUIN Question

Origin:
Department of Health. Using the Commissioning for Quality and Innovation (CQUIN) payment framework. Guidance on the new national goals 2012–13. London: Department of Health, 2012 [4].

Content:
"Have you been more forgetful in the past 12 months to the extent that it has significantly affected your life?"

© Springer Nature Switzerland AG 2020
A. J. Larner, *Manual of Screeners for Dementia*,
https://doi.org/10.1007/978-3-030-41636-2_2

Data:

Categorical:

- Yes: initiate "dementia risk assessment" (nature unspecified)
- No: no intervention.

Pragmatic studies:

Larner AJ. Metamemory: a construct with diagnostic utility in a cognitive disorders clinic? Int J Geriatr Psychiatry. 2018a;33:553–4 [8].

Results

For diagnosis of any cognitive impairment:

1. Demographics:

N	50
P = Prevalence of cognitive impairment (= pre-test probability)	0.48
Q = Level of the test = "Yes"	0.60

2. Paired measures of discrimination:

Sensitivity (Se), Specificity (Sp)	0.63, 0.42
PPV, NPV	0.50, 0.55
LR+, LR−	1.08, 0.89 (both slight)
CUI+, CUI-	0.31, 0.23 (both very poor)

3. Unitary measures of discrimination:

Accuracy	0.52
Y	0.05
PSI	0.05
SUI	0.54 (very poor)

4. Numbers needed:

To diagnose (NND)	20.0
To predict (NNP)	20.0
To misdiagnose (NNM)	2.08
Likelihood to be diagnosed or misdiagnosed (LDM = NNM/NND, NNM/NNP)	0.10, 0.10
For screening utility (NNSU)	1.85 (inadequate)

Conclusions:

This single-item cognitive screening question may be conceptualised as a test of metamemory. It is quick and easy to administer (<1 min) and easily categorised. It was answered affirmatively at high frequency both in this pragmatic study (Q = 0.60) and in a population of patients with epilepsy [1] who are known to be liable to subjective memory complaints.

All measures of discrimination and numbers needed were unfavourable, and less impressive than a patient-performance cognitive screening instrument (MACE) administered concurrently in the pragmatic study [8]. LDM metrics were <1, and SUI and NNSU values were poor and inadequate respectively.

The Dementia CQUIN question has now been "decommissioned". It stands as an example of how initiation of top-down (bureaucratic) policy without an evidence base may fail to achieve desired outcomes.

2.3 Subjective Memory Complaint (SMC) Likert Scale

Origin:

Paradise MB, Glozier NS, Naismith SL, Davenport TA, Hickie IB. Subjective memory complaints, vascular risk factors and psychological distress in the middle-aged: a cross-sectional study. BMC Psychiatry. 2011;11:108 [11].

Content:

A five-point Likert scale for subjective memory complaints (SMC). Participants are asked:

"In general, how would you rate your memory?"

with a choice of the following five responses:

- 1 = poor;
- 2 = fair;
- 3 = good;
- 4 = very good;
- 5 = excellent.

Data:

Although the Likert scale is an example of ordinal data (i.e. variables have ordered categories and the distances between the categories are not known; [12]), the interpretation used here is categorical and binary, i.e.:

- SMC+: those rating their memory as either fair or poor (2 or 1)
- SMC−: those rating their memory as good, very good, or excellent (3, 4, or 5).

Pragmatic studies:

Bharambe V, Larner AJ. Functional cognitive disorders: demographic and clinical features contribute to a positive diagnosis. Neurodegener Dis Manag. 2018;8:377–83 [3].

Larner AJ. Metamemory: a construct with diagnostic utility in a cognitive disorders clinic? Int J Geriatr Psychiatry. 2018a;33:553–4 [8].

Results

For diagnosis of no cognitive impairment:

1. Demographics:

N	130
P = Prevalence of cognitive impairment (= pre-test probability)	0.46
Q = Level of the test = SMC+	0.79

2. Paired measures of discrimination:

Sensitivity (Se), Specificity (Sp)	0.87, 0.30
PPV, NPV	0.59, 0.67
LR+, LR−	1.24 (slight), 0.43 (moderate)
CUI+, CUI−	0.52 (adequate), 0.20 (very poor)

3. Unitary measures of discrimination:

Accuracy	0.61
Y	0.17
PSI	0.26
SUI	0.72 (poor)

4. Numbers needed:

To diagnose (NND)	5.88
To predict (NNP)	3.85
To misdiagnose (NNM)	2.56
Likelihood to be diagnosed or misdiagnosed (LDM = NNM/NND, NNM/NNP)	0.44, 0.65
For screening utility (NNSU)	1.39 (inadequate)

Conclusions:

This single-item cognitive screening question may be conceptualised as a test of metamemory (other metamemory questionnaires are also based on Likert statements, e.g. the Metamemory in Adulthood Questionnaire; [5]). It is quick and easy to administer (<1 min) and easily categorised. It has been used as a measure of subjective memory complaint in studies of screening instruments for MCI [10].

The SMC Likert Scale was answered "fair" or "poor" (i.e. SMC+) at very high frequency in both these pragmatic studies (Q = 0.79) and also in a population of patients with epilepsy [2] who are known to be liable to subjective memory complaints.

Measures of discrimination show SMC Likert Scale to be a high sensitivity low specificity test (i.e. many false positives, few false negatives) for the absence of cognitive impairment, with resultant numbers needed metrics suggesting a poor balance in terms of misdiagnosis over diagnosis. LDM metrics were <1, and SUI and NNSU values were poor and inadequate respectively.

The SMC Likert Scale may be of merit in situations where clinicians are desirous of identifying all cases of cognitive impairment, accepting the risk of false positives. It may also have a role in screening for individuals with functional cognitive disorders, in whom disordered metamemory may be relevant to pathogenesis [9].

A similar, informant, 5-point Likert scale single screening question for dementia, SSQ-dementia, has also been developed [7].

The combination of SMC Likert Scale with a cognitive screening instrument (MACE) has also been examined (Sect. 12.2).

References

1. Aji BM, Larner AJ. Screening for dementia: is one simple question the answer? Clin Med. 2015;15:111–2.
2. Aji BM, Larner AJ. Screening for dementia: single yes/no question or Likert scale? Clin Med. 2017;17:93–4.
3. Bharambe V, Larner AJ. Functional cognitive disorders: demographic and clinical features contribute to a positive diagnosis. Neurodegener Dis Manag. 2018;8:377–83.
4. Department of Health. Using the commissioning for quality and innovation (CQUIN) payment framework. Guidance on the new national goals 2012–13. London: Department of Health;2012.
5. Dixon RA, Hultsch DF, Hertzog C. The metamemory in adulthood (MIA) questionnaire. Psychopharmacol Bull. 1988;24:671–88. Erratum in: Psychopharmacol Bull. 1989;25:157.
6. Hendry K, Hill E, Quinn TJ, Evans J, Stott DJ. Single screening questions for cognitive impairment in older people: a systematic review. Age Ageing. 2015a;44:322–6.
7. Hendry K, Quinn TJ, Evans JJ, Stott DJ. Informant single screening questions for delirium and dementia in acute care—a cross-sectional test accuracy pilot study. BMC Geriatr. 2015b;15:17.
8. Larner AJ. Metamemory: a construct with diagnostic utility in a cognitive disorders clinic? Int J Geriatr Psychiatry. 2018a;33:553–4.
9. Larner AJ. Dementia screening: a different proposal. Future Neurol. 2018b;13:177–9.
10. O'Caoimh R, Timmons S, Molloy DW. Screening for mild cognitive impairment: comparison of "MCI specific" screening instruments. J Alzheimers Dis. 2016;51:619–29.
11. Paradise MB, Glozier NS, Naismith SL, Davenport TA, Hickie IB. Subjective memory complaints, vascular risk factors and psychological distress in the middle-aged: a cross-sectional study. BMC Psychiatry. 2011;11:108.
12. Stevens SS. On the theory of scales of measurement. Science. 1946;103:677–80.

Chapter 3
Neurological Signs

3.1 Introduction

In addition to the standard neurological examination, which is undertaken in patients with cognitive complaints as for other neurological presentations, a number of "non-canonical" neurological signs have been described which may be of possible use in the assessment of patients with cognitive complaints [22, 24]. The evaluation of these signs is described here.

It should be noted that the neurological signs discussed here have been examined in a high prevalence secondary care setting (P for cognitive impairment of around 0.3–0.6). For the utility of these signs in primary care and community settings with lower disease prevalence, calculations may be undertaken using standard equations (Sect. 1.3.2, Eqs. 1.1 and 1.2).

3.2 Attended Alone (AA) Sign

Origin:
Larner AJ. "Who came with you?" A diagnostic observation in patients with memory problems? J Neurol Neurosurg Psychiatry. 2005;76:1739 [19].

Larner AJ. "Attended alone" sign: validity and reliability for the exclusion of dementia. Age Ageing. 2009;38:476–8 [20].

Content:
Attended alone (AA) sign is an indicator of the absence of cognitive impairment, or conversely the presence of cognitive health or wellbeing.

© Springer Nature Switzerland AG 2020
A. J. Larner, *Manual of Screeners for Dementia*,
https://doi.org/10.1007/978-3-030-41636-2_3

Data:

Categorical:

- AA sign present: the patient attends the clinic consultation alone
- AA sign absent: patient attends clinic consultation accompanied (attended with sign, see Sect. 3.3)

Pragmatic studies:

Larner AJ. Screening utility of the "attended alone" sign for subjective memory impairment. Alzheimer Dis Assoc Disord. 2014b;28:364–5 [23].

Results

(A) For diagnosis of no cognitive impairment:

1. Demographics:

N	726
P = Prevalence of cognitive impairment (= pre-test probability)	0.32
Q = Level of the test	0.34

2. Paired measures of discrimination:

Sensitivity (Se), Specificity (Sp)	0.93, 0.45
PPV, NPV	0.47, 0.93
LR+, LR−	1.70 (slight), 0.14 (large)
CUI+, CUI−	0.44, 0.42 (both poor)

3. Unitary measures of discrimination:

Accuracy	0.61
Y	0.38
PSI	0.40
SUI	0.86 (poor)

4. Numbers needed:

To diagnose (NND)	2.63
To predict (NNP)	2.50
To misdiagnose (NNM)	2.56

Likelihood to be diagnosed or misdiagnosed (LDM = NNM/NND, NNM/NNP)	0.97, 1.02
For screening utility (NNSU)	1.16 (inadequate)

(B) For diagnosis of no dementia:

1. Demographics:

N	726
P = Prevalence of cognitive impairment (= pre-test probability)	0.32
Q = Level of the test	0.34

2. Paired measures of discrimination:

Sensitivity (Se), Specificity (Sp)	1.00, 0.45
PPV, NPV	0.48, 1.00
LR+, LR−	1.82 (slight), 0 (very large)
CUI+, CUI−	0.48, 0.45 (both poor)

3. Unitary measures of discrimination:

Accuracy	0.64
Y	0.45
PSI	0.48
SUI	0.93 (poor)

4. Numbers needed:

To diagnose (NND)	2.22
To predict (NNP)	2.08
To misdiagnose (NNM)	2.78
Likelihood to be diagnosed or misdiagnosed (LDM = NNM/NND, NNM/NNP)	1.25, 1.37
For screening utility (NNSU)	1.08 (inadequate)

Conclusions:

This non-canonical neurological sign is quick and easy to observe and categorise (<1 min). Despite instructions to patients to attend with a reliable informant for the purpose of collateral history taking, a significant number attend alone (Q = 0.34).

The evidence from pragmatic studies is that the attended alone sign is very sensitive for the absence of significant cognitive impairment (dementia and MCI) with large NPV and LR−. However, LDM metrics were ≈1, and SUI and NNSU values were poor and inadequate respectively. Patient gender does not appear to influence the measures of discrimination [1]. A prospective study examining the screening metrics of AA sign in a large cohort (N > 1200) is due to report in 2020 (Larner AJ. Postgrad Med. 2020 Mar 5. https://doi.org/10.1080/00325481.2020.17 39416. [Epub ahead of print]).

In a separate study, the attended alone sign was found to be of possible value in the positive diagnosis of functional cognitive disorders [4, 5].

The findings of high sensitivity and NPV and large LR− have been reported in an independent study of AA sign from a general psychology clinic in the USA [34]. Attended alone sign has been mentioned in didactic [10, p. 518] and popular neurological texts [33, p. 34,267]. Use of this simple behavioural index has been contrasted with current clinical practice using more sophisticated investigation modalities in MCI and Alzheimer's disease [17].

3.3   Attended with (AW) Sign

Origin:
Soysal P, Usarel C, Ispirli G, Isik AT. Attended with and head-turning sign can be clinical markers of cognitive impairment in older adults. Int Psychogeriatr. 2017;29:1763–9 [32].

Content:
Attended with (AW) sign is an indicator of the presence of cognitive impairment. It has sometimes been referred to as the "negative attended alone sign (NAAS)".

Data:
Categorical:

- AW sign present: patient attends clinic consultation accompanied by an informant
- AW sign absent: patient attends clinic consultation alone (attended alone sign, see Sect. 3.2)

Pragmatic studies:
Larner AJ. Screening utility of the "attended alone" sign for subjective memory impairment. Alzheimer Dis Assoc Disord. 2014b;28:364–5 [23].

Williamson JC, Larner AJ. Attended with and head-turning sign can be clinical markers of cognitive impairment in older adults. Int Psychogeriatr. 2018;30:1569 [35].

Results
For diagnosis of any cognitive impairment:

1. Demographics:

N	726
P = Prevalence of cognitive impairment (= pre-test probability)	0.32
Q = Level of the test	0.66

2. Paired measures of discrimination:

Sensitivity (Se), Specificity (Sp)	0.93, 0.47
PPV, NPV	0.45, 0.93
LR+, LR−	1.74 (slight), 0.15 (large)
CUI+, CUI−	0.42, 0.44 (both poor)

3. Unitary measures of discrimination:

Accuracy	0.61
Y	0.40
PSI	0.38
SUI	0.86 (poor)

4. Numbers needed:

To diagnose (NND)	2.50
To predict (NNP)	2.63
To misdiagnose (NNM)	2.56
Likelihood to be diagnosed or misdiagnosed (LDM = NNM/NND, NNM/NNP)	1.02, 0.97
For screening utility (NNSU)	1.16 (inadequate)

Conclusions:
This non-canonical neurological sign is, like its converse, the attended alone sign (Sect. 3.2), quick and easy to observe and categorise (<1 min), and is very frequently seen (Q = 0.66).

The evidence from pragmatic studies is that the attended with sign is very sensitive for the presence of significant cognitive impairment (dementia and MCI). However, LDM metrics were ≈1, and SUI and NNSU values were inadequate.

A prospective study examining the screening metrics of AW sign in a large cohort (N > 1200) is due to report in 2020 (Larner AJ. Postgrad Med. 2020 Mar 5. https://doi.org/10.1080/00325481.2020.1739416. [Epub ahead of print]). A preliminary finding from this study is that for the subgroup of patients attending the clinic with two or more informants (prevalence = 0.1 of AW), termed the "AW2+ sign", positive predictive value for any cognitive impairment is higher (0.85) than for all AW (0.61).

The attended with sign has also been incorporated in the Triple Test [16, 18] (see Sect. 12.3).

3.4 Head Turning Sign (HTS)

Origin:
Bouchard RW, Rossor MN. Typical clinical features. In: Gauthier S (ed.). Clinical diagnosis and management of Alzheimer's disease. London: Martin Dunitz; 1996, pp. 35–50 [7, p. 37].

Content:
Head turning sign (HTS) is an indicator of the presence of cognitive impairment. HTS may be variously operationalised, but is most simply based on the clinician's observation that the patient turns her/his head away from the examining interlocutor towards an accompanying person during the history taking section of the clinical assessment. Others have operationalised the sign on the basis of head turning during administration of cognitive screeners [11], but this goes against widely applied policy recommendations to exclude third persons during cognitive testing [28].

Data:
Categorical:

- HTS present: patient turns head away from the interlocutor and towards the accompanying person(s) when first invited to describe symptoms (e.g. "Tell me about the problems you are having with your memory") or when specifically asked about them (e.g. "What problems are you having with your memory?" or "Can you give me an example of how your memory lets you down?").
- HTS absent: patient does not turn head to interlocutor.

Pragmatic studies:
Ghadiri-Sani M, Larner AJ. Head turning sign for diagnosis of dementia and mild cognitive impairment: a revalidation. J Neurol Neurosurg Psychiatry. 2013;84:e2 [12].

Larner AJ. Head turning sign: pragmatic utility in clinical diagnosis of cognitive impairment. J Neurol Neurosurg Psychiatry. 2012;83:852–3 [21].

Williamson JC, Larner AJ. Attended with and head-turning sign can be clinical markers of cognitive impairment in older adults. Int Psychogeriatr. 2018;30:1569 [35].

Results

For diagnosis of any cognitive impairment:

1. Demographics:

N	246
P = Prevalence of cognitive impairment (= pre-test probability)	0.63
Q = Level of the test	0.43

2. Paired measures of discrimination:

Sensitivity (Se), Specificity (Sp)	0.65, 0.95
PPV, NPV	0.95, 0.61
LR+, LR−	11.9 (very large), 0.37 (moderate)
CUI+, CUI−	0.62, 0.58 (both adequate)

3. Unitary measures of discrimination:

Accuracy	0.76
Y	0.60
PSI	0.56
SUI	1.20 (adequate)

4. Numbers needed:

To diagnose (NND)	1.67
To predict (NNP)	1.79
To misdiagnose (NNM)	4.17
Likelihood to be diagnosed or misdiagnosed (LDM = NNM/NND, NNM/NNP)	2.50, 2.33
For screening utility (NNSU)	0.83 (adequate)

Conclusions:

This non-canonical neurological sign is quick and easy to observe and categorise (<1 min).

In these pragmatic studies, HTS was seen with moderate frequency (Q = 0.43) and was more specific than sensitive, with high PPV and LR+. The unitary (LDM, SUI, NNSU) and number needed metrics were reasonable, and more favourable than those of the other non-canonical signs considered in this chapter [24, 25].

However, these findings differ from those of Soysal et al. [32] who reported HTS to have high sensitivity and NPV for cognitive impairment. It is possible that methodological and cultural factors may have contributed to these discrepancies. For example, HTS was found in many more normals in the Soysal study than in the pragmatic experience reported here, perhaps related to an older age structure of the study population and a higher percentage of female participants [13]. Re-analysis of the pragmatic data indicated the possible involvement of behavioural factors, as HTS was found to have greater diagnostic accuracy in female patients [1].

Methods to scale HTS have been suggested [9, 11], raising the possibility of using ordinal data to evaluate the sign in future studies [13].

The head turning sign has also been incorporated in the Triple Test [16, 18] (see Sect. 12.3), and has been mentioned in some neurological texts, both didactic [3, p. 65; 10, p. 517; 15, p. 107; 31, p. 326] and popular [33, p. 41]. Use of this simple behavioural index has been contrasted with current clinical practice using more sophisticated investigation modalities in MCI and Alzheimer's disease [17].

3.5 Applause Sign

Origin:
Dubois B, Slachevsky A, Pillon B, Beato R, Villalponda JM, Litvan I. "Applause sign" helps to discriminate PSP from FTD and PD. Neurology. 2005;64:2132–3 [8].

Content:
Applause sign is an indicator of the presence of cognitive impairment.

Data:
Categorical:

- Applause sign present: when asked to clap three times (examiner may demonstrate this to the patient), the patient claps more than three times
- Applause sign absent: patient claps three times, as requested or demonstrated

Pragmatic studies:
Bonello M, Larner AJ. Applause sign: screening utility for dementia and cognitive impairment. Postgrad Med. 2016;128:250–3 [6].

Results
(A) For diagnosis of any cognitive impairment:

1. Demographics:

N	275
P = Prevalence of cognitive impairment (= pre-test probability)	0.45
Q = Level of the test	0.22

2. Paired measures of discrimination:

Sensitivity (Se), Specificity (Sp)	0.36, 0.89
PPV, NPV	0.72, 0.63
LR+, LR−	3.18 (moderate), 0.72 (slight)
CUI+, CUI−	0.26 (very poor), 0.59 (adequate)

3. Unitary measures of discrimination:

Accuracy	0.65
Y	0.25
PSI	0.35
SUI	0.85 (poor)

4. Numbers needed:

To diagnose (NND)	4.00
To predict (NNP)	2.86
To misdiagnose (NNM)	2.86
Likelihood to be diagnosed or misdiagnosed (LDM = NNM/NND, NNM/NNP)	0.72, 1.00
For screening utility (NNSU)	1.18 (inadequate)

(B) For diagnosis of dementia:

1. Demographics:

N	275
P = Prevalence of cognitive impairment (= pre-test probability)	0.45
Q = Level of the test	0.22

2. Paired measures of discrimination:

Sensitivity (Se), Specificity (Sp)	0.54, 0.85
PPV, NPV	0.46, 0.89
LR+, LR−	3.59 (moderate), 0.54 (slight)
CUI+, CUI−	0.25 (very poor), 0.75 (good)

3. Unitary measures of discrimination:

Accuracy	0.79
Y	0.39
PSI	0.35
SUI	1.00 (adequate)

4. Numbers needed:

To diagnose (NND)	2.56
To predict (NNP)	2.86
To misdiagnose (NNM)	4.76
Likelihood to be diagnosed or misdiagnosed (LDM = NNM/NND, NNM/NNP)	1.86, 1.66
For screening utility (NNSU)	1.00 (adequate)

Conclusions:
This non-canonical neurological sign is quick and easy to perform and categorise (<1 min).

The applause sign has a relatively low prevalence (Q = 0.22), and in this pragmatic study it was found to be more specific than sensitive, with high PPV and LR+, confirming the findings of a prior (smaller) study [2], suggesting the sign is reproducible. The unitary (LDM, SUI, NNSU) and number needed metrics were not as good as for the head turning sign (Sect. 3.4).

Methods to scale the applause sign have been suggested [26]: the "applause sign score" is inversely related to the number of claps and raises the possibility of using ordinal data to evaluate the sign in future studies. Applause sign may be independent of disease severity in Alzheimer's disease [27].

The applause sign has also been incorporated in the Triple Test [16, 18] (see Sect. 12.3).

3.6 *La maladie du petit papier*

Origin:
The origin of the term is uncertain, but may possibly derive from Charcot's clinics in 19th century Paris.

Content:
La maladie du petit papier is an indicator of the absence of cognitive impairment.

Data:
Categorical:

- Sign present: patient presents or reads from a written or typed (paper, iPad) list of symptoms at time of consultation
- Sign absent: patient does not bring a written list

Pragmatic studies:
Bharambe V, Larner AJ. Functional cognitive disorders: demographic and clinical features contribute to a positive diagnosis. Neurodegener Dis Manag. 2018b;8:377–83 [5].

Randall A, Larner AJ. *La maladie du petit papier*: a sign of functional cognitive disorder? Int J Geriatr Psychiatry. 2018;33:800 [30].

Results
For diagnosis of any cognitive impairment:

1. Demographics:

N	258
P = Prevalence of cognitive impairment (= pre-test probability)	0.41
Q = Level of the test	0.05

2. Paired measures of discrimination:

Sensitivity (Se), Specificity (Sp)	0.07, 0.98
PPV, NPV	0.85, 0.43
LR+, LR−	3.90 (moderate), 0.94 (slight)
CUI+, CUI−	0.06 (very poor), 0.42 (poor)

3. Unitary measures of discrimination:

Accuracy	0.45
Y	0.05
PSI	0.28
SUI	0.48 (very poor)

4. Numbers needed:

To diagnose (NND)	20.0
To predict (NNP)	3.57
To misdiagnose (NNM)	1.82
Likelihood to be diagnosed or misdiagnosed (LDM = NNM/NND, NNM/NNP)	0.09, 0.51
For screening utility (NNSU)	2.08 (inadequate)

Conclusions:

This non-canonical neurological sign is quick and easy to observe and categorise (<1 min). *La maladie du petit papier* is a very low prevalence sign (Q = 0.05) although this is higher than the frequency observed in general neurology clinics [29].

The overall metrics are less favourable than for the other non-canonical neurological signs, including the unitary metrics (LDM, SUI, NNSU), but the specificity, PPV, and LR+ are worthy of note, suggesting this observation is helpful in ruling out cognitive impairment. There may also, of course, be qualitative value in paying attention to the matters of sufficient concern to patients to prompt them to write them down [14].

La maladie du petit papier has been mentioned in a popular neurological text [33, p. 220].

References

1. Abernethy Holland AJ, Larner AJ. Effects of gender on two clinical signs (attended alone and head turning) of use in the diagnosis of cognitive complaints. J Neurol Sci. 2013a;333:e295–6
2. Abernethy Holland AJ, Larner AJ. Applause sign: diagnostic utility in a cognitive function clinic. J Neurol Sci. 2013b;333:e292.
3. Alpert JN. The neurologic diagnosis. A practical bedside approach. 2nd ed. New York: Springer; 2019.
4. Bharambe V, Larner AJ. Functional cognitive disorders: memory clinic study. Prog Neurol Psychiatry. 2018a;22(3):19–22.

5. Bharambe V, Larner AJ. Functional cognitive disorders: demographic and clinical features contribute to a positive diagnosis. Neurodegener Dis Manag. 2018b;8:377–83.

6. Bonello M, Larner AJ. Applause sign: screening utility for dementia and cognitive impairment. Postgrad Med. 2016;128:250–3.

7. Bouchard RW, Rossor MN. Typical clinical features. In: Gauthier S (ed.). Clinical diagnosis and management of Alzheimer's disease. London: Martin Dunitz; 1996, pp. 35–50 (at p. 37).

8. Dubois B, Slachevsky A, Pillon B, Beato R, Villalponda JM, Litvan I. "Applause sign" helps to discriminate PSP from FTD and PD. Neurology. 2005;64:2132–3.

9. Duraes J, Tabuas-Pereira M, Araujo R, et al. The head turning sign in dementia and mild cognitive impairment: its relationship to cognition, behavior, and cerebrospinal fluid biomarkers. Dement Geriatr Cogn Disord. 2018;46:42–9.

10. Ellajosyula R. Clinical approach and classification of dementia syndromes. In: Mukherjee A, editor. IAN textbook of neurology. New Delhi: Jaypee; 2018. p. 515–21.

11. Fukui T, Yamazaki R, Kinno R. Can the "Head-Turning Sign" be a clinical marker of Alzheimer's disease? Dement Geriatr Cogn Disord Extra. 2011;1:310–7.

12. Ghadiri-Sani M, Larner AJ. Head turning sign for diagnosis of dementia and mild cognitive impairment: a revalidation. J Neurol Neurosurg Psychiatry. 2013;84:e2.

13. Ghadiri-Sani M, Larner AJ. Head turning sign. J R Coll Physicians Edinb. 2019;49:323–6.

14. Grover S. Don't dismiss the little notes that patients bring. BMJ. 2015;350:h20.

15. Hodges JR. Cognitive assessment for clinicians, 3rd ed. Oxford: Oxford University Press, 2018.

16. Isik AT, Soysal P, Kaya D, Usarel C. Triple test, a diagnostic observation, can detect cognitive impairment in older adults. Psychogeriatrics. 2018;18:98–105.

17. Judge D, Roberts J, Khandker RK, Ambegaonkar B, Black CM. Physician practice patterns associated with diagnostic evaluation of patients with suspected mild cognitive impairment and Alzheimer's disease. Int J Alzheimers Dis. 2019;2019:4942562.

18. Koc Okudur S, Dokuzlar O, Kaya D, Soysal P, Isik AT. Triple Test plus Rapid Cognitive Screening Test: a combination of clinical signs and a tool for cognitive assessment in older adults. Diagnostics (Basel). 2019;9:E97.

19. Larner AJ. "Who came with you?" A diagnostic observation in patients with memory problems? J Neurol Neurosurg Psychiatry. 2005;76:1739.

20. Larner AJ. "Attended alone" sign: validity and reliability for the exclusion of dementia. Age Ageing. 2009;38:476–8.

21. Larner AJ. Head turning sign: pragmatic utility in clinical diagnosis of cognitive impairment. J Neurol Neurosurg Psychiatry. 2012;83:852–3.

22. Larner AJ. Neurological signs of possible diagnostic value in the cognitive disorders clinic. Pract Neurol. 2014a;14:332–5.

23. Larner AJ. Screening utility of the "attended alone" sign for subjective memory impairment. Alzheimer Dis Assoc Disord. 2014b;28:364–5.

24. Larner AJ. Number needed to diagnose (NND), predict (NNP), or misdiagnose (NNM): useful metrics for non-canonical signs of cognitive status? Dement Geriatr Cogn Dis Extra. 2018;8:321–7.

25. Larner AJ. New unitary metrics for dementia test accuracy studies. Prog Neurol Psychiatry. 2019;23(3):21–5.

26. Luzzi S, Fabi K, Pesallaccia M, Silvestrini M, Provinciali L. Applause sign: is it really specific for Parkinsonian disorders? Evidence from cortical dementias. J Neurol Neurosurg Psychiatry. 2011;82:830–3.

27. Luzzi S, Fabi K, Pesallaccia M, Silvestrini M, Provinciali L. Applause sign in Alzheimer's disease: relationships to cognitive profile and severity of illness. J Neurol. 2013;260:172–5.

28. Members of the Task Force. Policy statement on the presence of third party observers in neuropsychological assessments. Clin Neuropsychol. 2001;15:433–9.

29. Randall A, Larner AJ. La maladie du petit papier: quantitative survey, clinical significance. J Neurol Neurosurg Psychiatry. 2016;87:e1.

30. Randall A, Larner AJ. *La maladie du petit papier*: a sign of functional cognitive disorder? Int J Geriatr Psychiatry. 2018;33:800.
31. Scheltens P. Dementia. In: Kuks JBM, Snoek JW, editors. Textbook of clinical neurology. Houten: Bohn Stafleu van Loghum; 2018.
32. Soysal P, Usarel C, Ispirli G, Isik AT. Attended with and head-turning sign can be clinical markers of cognitive impairment in older adults. Int Psychogeriatr. 2017;29:1763–9.
33. Tubridy N. Just one more question. Stories from a life in neurology. London: Penguin Ireland; 2019.
34. Tyson BT, Cabrera L, Scriven E, Larios C, Reilly E, Kearns L. The diagnostic utility of the "attended alone" sign for dementia in patients presenting for neuropsychological evaluation. J Neuroinflamm Neurodegener Dis. 2019;3(1):100010.
35. Williamson JC, Larner AJ. Attended with and head-turning sign can be clinical markers of cognitive impairment in older adults. Int Psychogeriatr. 2018;30:1569.

Chapter 4
Cognitive Screeners (1): Brief Patient-Performance Scales (<5 Min)

4.1 Introduction

Patient-performance scales are the most commonly applied cognitive screeners. A large range of tests is available (see, for example [7, 16]). These vary in their exact length, item content, cognitive domains examined, and hence in time to administer.

In this chapter pragmatic studies of patient-performance scales which ordinarily take <5 min to administer are examined. These usually comprise 3–8 items, and are suitable for use in primary care and other settings where assessment is time-limited. A number of the screeners discussed here have been subjected to analysis using the new unitary metrics of LDM, SUI and NNSU [19, 20].

Clock drawing is usually included amongst brief patient-performance scales, and there is a large literature on various forms of administration and scoring [22]. Although not examined in isolation here, clock drawing does feature as a component of Mini-Cog and Codex (Sects. 4.2 and 4.3) as well as other screeners (e.g. Montreal Cognitive Assessment, Addenbrooke's Examinations; Chap. 6).

Hodkinson's Abbreviated Mental Test Score (AMTS), one of the earliest cognitive screeners to be described [13], also falls within this category. Several versions are now described [25], but none has been examined in this clinic, although encountered in patients referred from primary care settings [8].

Another very short screening test is the Rapid Cognitive Screen which, like Mini-Cog and Codex, incorporates word recall and clock drawing [23]. A test designed to identify cases of MCI, the Quick Mild Cognitive Impairment screen (Q*mci*) may be completed in 3–5 minutes [24].

Longer screening tests and informant scales form the subject of following chapters (Chaps. 5, 6 and 7).

© Springer Nature Switzerland AG 2020
A. J. Larner, *Manual of Screeners for Dementia*,
https://doi.org/10.1007/978-3-030-41636-2_4

4.2   Mini-Cog

Origin:
Borson S, Scanlan J, Brush M, Vitiliano P, Dokmak A. The Mini-Cog: a cognitive "vital signs" measure for dementia screening in multi-lingual elderly. Int J Geriatr Psychiatry. 2000;15:1021–7 [5].

Content:
A three word recall task (scored 0–3) and a clock drawing task (scored abnormal-normal).

Data:
Categorical: "dementia" or "no dementia".

In the standard scoring system, a score of zero or three on the word recall task leads to categorization as "dementia" or "no dementia" respectively; for the intermediate scores on word recall, 1 or 2, performance on the clock drawing task is then taken into account: if normal or abnormal the patient is categorized as "no dementia" or "dementia", respectively.

Pragmatic studies:
Larner AJ. Mini-Cog versus Codex (cognitive disorders examination): is there a difference? Dement Neuropsychol. 2020:accepted [21].

Results
(A) For diagnosis of dementia:

1. Demographics:

N	162
P = Prevalence of dementia (= pre-test probability)	0.27
Q = Level of the test	0.43

2. Paired measures of discrimination:

Sensitivity (Se), Specificity (Sp)	0.87, 0.74
PPV, NPV	0.56, 0.95
LR+, LR−	3.37 (moderate), 0.15 (large)
CUI+, CUI−	0.498 (adequate), 0.70 (good)

3. Unitary measures of discrimination:

Accuracy	0.78
Y	0.51

| PSI | 0.56 |
| SUI | 1.19 (adequate) |

4. Numbers needed:

To diagnose (NND)	1.49
To predict (NNP)	1.72
To misdiagnose (NNM)	4.50
Likelihood to be diagnosed or misdiagnosed (LDM = NNM/NND, NNM/NNP)	3.02, 2.61
For screening utility (NNSU)	0.84 (adequate)

(B) For diagnosis of MCI versus no cognitive impairment:

1. Demographics:

N	118
P = Prevalence of mild cognitive impairment (= pre-test probability)	0.22
Q = Level of the test	0.26

2. Paired measures of discrimination:

Sensitivity (Se), Specificity (Sp)	0.69, 0.86
PPV, NPV	0.58, 0.91
LR+, LR−	4.90 (moderate), 0.36 (moderate)
CUI+, CUI−	0.40 (poor), 0.78 (good)

3. Unitary measures of discrimination:

Accuracy	0.82
Y	0.55
PSI	0.49
SUI	1.18 (adequate)

4. Numbers needed:

| To diagnose (NND) | 1.82 |
| To predict (NNP) | 2.04 |

To misdiagnose (NNM)	5.62
Likelihood to be diagnosed or misdiagnosed (LDM = NNM/NND, NNM/NNP)	3.09, 2.75
For screening utility (NNSU)	0.85 (adequate)

Conclusions:

The Mini-Cog has been widely studied, in community [11], primary care [26], and secondary care settings [9], although systematic reviews have been unable to make firm conclusions about test utility for diagnosis of dementia.

In this patient cohort, test metrics suggested utility for dementia diagnosis (high sensitivity and NPV, large LR−). The unitary metrics showed good LDM and adequate SUI and NNSU. However metrics for MCI were less encouraging. Nevertheless, in a weighted comparison with Codex (Sect. 4.3), Mini-Cog had net benefit screening for MCI as well as being essentially equivalent screening for dementia.

Utility of Mini-Cog in primary care settings might be examined using the method of cross-classifying primary care Mini-Cog test scores with secondary care reference diagnoses, as reported for 6CIT (Sect. 4.4; [10]) and MMSE (Sect. 5.2; [18]).

4.3   Codex (Cognitive Disorders Examination)

Origin:

Belmin J, Pariel-Madjlessi S, Surun P, Bentot C, Feteanu D, Lefebvre des Noettes V, et al. The cognitive disorders examination (Codex) is a reliable 3-minute test for detection of dementia in the elderly (validation study in 323 subjects). Presse Med. 2007a;36:1183–90 [3].

Belmin J, Oasi C, Folio P, Pariel-Madjlessi S. Codex, un test ultra-rapide pour le repérage des démences chez les sujets âgés. Revue Geriatr. 2007b;32:627–31 [4].

Content:

A two-step decision tree (Fig. 4.1) incorporating the three-word recall and spatial orientation components from the MMSE (Sect. 5.2) along with a simplified clock drawing test (sCDT), which takes around three minutes to perform.

Data:

Categorical, with differing probabilities of dementia: A = very low, B = low, C = high, D − very high (Fig. 4.1).

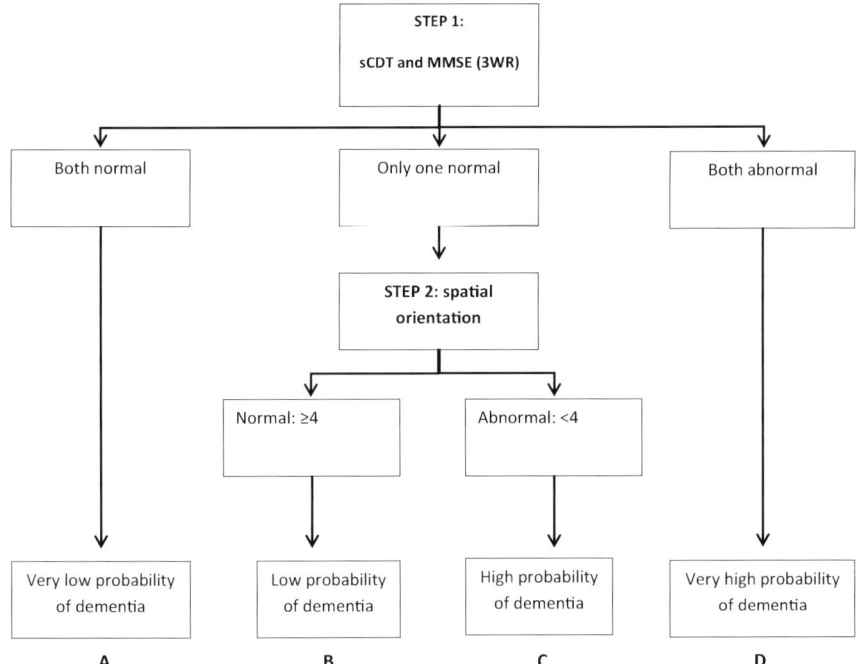

Fig. 4.1 Codex decision tree

Pragmatic studies:

Larner AJ. Codex (cognitive disorders examination) for the detection of dementia and mild cognitive impairment. Codex pour la détection de la démence et du mild cognitive impairment. Presse Med. 2013;42:e425–8 [14].

Ziso B, Larner AJ. Codex (cognitive disorders examination) for the detection of dementia and mild cognitive impairment: diagnostic utility. J Neurol Neurosurg Psychiatry. 2013;84:e2 [28].

Results
(A) For diagnosis of dementia, categories C and D (from index study):

1. Demographics:

N	162
P = Prevalence of dementia (= pre-test probability)	0.27
Q = Level of the test	0.35

2. Paired measures of discrimination:

Sensitivity (Se), Specificity (Sp)	0.84, 0.82
PPV, NPV	0.63, 0.93
LR+, LR−	4.74 (moderate), 0.20 (moderate)
CUI+, CUI−	0.53 (adequate), 0.77 (good)

3. Unitary measures of discrimination:

Accuracy	0.83
Y	0.66
PSI	0.56
SUI	1.30 (good)

4. Numbers needed:

To diagnose (NND)	1.52
To predict (NNP)	1.79
To misdiagnose (NNM)	5.88
Likelihood to be diagnosed or misdiagnosed (LDM = NNM/NND, NNM/NNP)	3.88, 3.29
For screening utility (NNSU)	0.77 (good)

(B) For diagnosis of any cognitive impairment, categories C and D (from index study):

1. Demographics:

N	162
P = Prevalence of any cognitive impairment (= pre-test probability)	0.44
Q = Level of the test	0.35

2. Paired measures of discrimination:

Sensitivity (Se), Specificity (Sp)	0.68, 0.91
PPV, NPV	0.86, 0.78
LR+, LR−	7.66 (large), 0.35 (moderate)
CUI+, CUI−	0.59 (adequate), 0.71 (good)

3. Unitary measures of discrimination:

Accuracy	0.81
Y	0.59
PSI	0.64
SUI	1.30 (good)

4. Numbers needed:

To diagnose (NND)	1.69
To predict (NNP)	1.56
To misdiagnose (NNM)	5.26
Likelihood to be diagnosed or misdiagnosed (LDM = NNM/NND, NNM/NNP)	3.11, 3.37
For screening utility (NNSU)	0.77 (good)

(C) For diagnosis of MCI versus no cognitive impairment, categories C and D (from index study):

1. Demographics:

N	118
P = Prevalence of mild cognitive impairment (= pre-test probability)	0.22
Q = Level of the test	0.17

2. Paired measures of discrimination:

Sensitivity (Se), Specificity (Sp)	0.42, 0.90
PPV, NPV	0.55, 0.85
LR+, LR−	4.32 (moderate), 0.64 (slight)
CUI+, CUI−	0.23 (very poor), 0.76 (good)

3. Unitary measures of discrimination:

Accuracy	0.80
Y	0.32
PSI	0.40
SUI	0.99 (adequate)

4. Numbers needed:

To diagnose (NND)	3.13
To predict (NNP)	2.50
To misdiagnose (NNM)	5.00
Likelihood to be diagnosed or misdiagnosed (LDM = NNM/NND, NNM/NNP)	1.60, 2.00
For screening utility (NNSU)	1.01 (adequate)

Conclusions:
Despite its ease of use (2–3 min to administer and score) and good metrics for dementia diagnosis, Codex has found rather limited application, mostly within France (e.g., [27]; see [2] for an exception). This may perhaps result from competition in the field of short variants of MMSE [17], but more likely due to limitations in using decision trees and categorical data derived therefrom as opposed to use of standard cognitive screening instruments generating quantitative data.

Data reported from this pragmatic study suggested better screening performance for dementia (high sensitivity and specificity) than for MCI (loss of sensitivity). LDM, SUI and NNSU were all encouraging for dementia diagnosis, but less so for MCI.

Modifications to Codex attempting to improve its sensitivity for diagnosis of MCI, based on more stringent tests of delayed recall extracted from studies of other cognitive screening instruments (specifically Montreal Cognitive Assessment and Free-Cog; Sects. 6.5 and 6.7 respectively) failed to improve upon the original Codex test metrics [29]. In a weighted comparison with Mini-Cog (Sect. 4.2), Codex was essentially equivalent screening for dementia but less good screening for MCI [21].

4.4   Six-Item Cognitive Impairment Test (6CIT)

Origin:
Brooke P, Bullock R. Validation of a 6 item cognitive impairment test with a view to primary care usage. Int J Geriatr Psychiatry. 1999;14:936–40 [6].

Content:
The Six-Item Cognitive Impairment Test (6CIT) is a brief (2–3 minute) cognitive screener which covers a limited number of cognitive domains.

Orientation (year, month, time)	10
Calculation (20–1, months backwards)	8

Memory recall (5 item name and address)	10
(NB negatively scored, i.e. higher score = worse performance)	
Total score	**28**

Data:

Quantitative, discrete, ordinal. Score range 28–0, impaired to normal (i.e. negatively scored). Scores are classified to aid test interpretation, e.g.:

- 0–4: "normal cognition"
- 5–9: "questionable impairment"
- $\geq$10: "suggesting impairment consistent with dementia and requiring further evaluation"

Another classification considers scores of 0–7 normal and $\geq$8 significant.

Pragmatic studies:

Abdel-Aziz K, Larner AJ. Six-Item Cognitive Impairment Test (6CIT) for detection of dementia and cognitive impairment. Int Psychogeriatr. 2015;27:991–7 [1].

Results

(A) For diagnosis of dementia, cut-off $\leq$9/28 (from index study):

1. Demographics:

N	245
P = Prevalence of dementia (= pre-test probability)	0.20
Q = Level of the test	0.37

2. Paired measures of discrimination:

Sensitivity (Se), Specificity (Sp)	0.88, 0.78
PPV, NPV	0.49, 0.96
LR+, LR−	4.00 (moderate), 0.16 (large)
CUI+, CUI−	0.43 (poor), 0.75 (good)

3. Unitary measures of discrimination:

| Accuracy | 0.80 |
| Y | 0.66 |

| PSI | 0.45 |
| SUI | 1.18 (adequate) |

4. Numbers needed:

To diagnose (NND)	1.51
To predict (NNP)	2.22
To misdiagnose (NNM)	5.00
Likelihood to be diagnosed or misdiagnosed (LDM = NNM/NND, NNM/NNP)	3.30, 2.25
For screening utility (NNSU)	0.85 (adequate)

(B) For diagnosis of mild cognitive impairment, cut-off ≤4/28 (from index study):

1. Demographics:

N	197
P = Prevalence of mild cognitive impairment (= pre-test probability)	0.27
Q = Level of the test	0.42

2. Paired measures of discrimination:

Sensitivity (Se), Specificity (Sp)	0.66, 0.70
PPV, NPV	0.53, 0.80
LR+, LR−	2.19 (moderate), 0.49 (moderate)
CUI+, CUI−	0.35 (very poor), 0.56 (adequate)

3. Unitary measures of discrimination:

Accuracy	0.69
Y	0.36
PSI	0.33
SUI	0.91 (poor)

4. Numbers needed:

| To diagnose (NND) | 2.78 |
| To predict (NNP) | 3.03 |

To misdiagnose (NNM)	3.23
Likelihood to be diagnosed or misdiagnosed (LDM = NNM/NND, NNM/NNP)	1.16, 1.06
For screening utility (NNSU)	1.10 (inadequate)

Conclusions:

In the pragmatic secondary care study, 6CIT had both high sensitivity and specificity and good unitary metrics (LDM, SUI and NNSU) for dementia diagnosis but not for MCI. Re-interrogating the study data using a different, higher, cut-off ($\geq 8/28$) showed greater sensitivity and lower specificity for dementia diagnosis but with the inverse pattern for MCI diagnosis [15].

6CIT was originally designed for use in primary care although a review of the literature [12] found few studies originating from this setting. Nevertheless 6CIT scores were often mentioned in referrals from primary care to dedicated cognitive disorders clinic [8]. Using 6CIT results from patients tested in primary care prior to (reference standard) diagnosis in secondary care showed more modest results for both 6CIT sensitivity and specificity [10] than in the pragmatic secondary care study analysed here.

References

1. Abdel-Aziz K, Larner AJ. Six-Item Cognitive Impairment Test (6CIT) for detection of dementia and cognitive impairment. Int Psychogeriatr. 2015;27:991–7.
2. Avgerinou C, Koufogianni K, Solini-Kosti E, Belmin J. Validation of the Greek translation of the Cognitive Disorders Examination (Codex) for the detection of dementia in primary care. Ann Hellenic Med. 2017;34:334–42.
3. Belmin J, Pariel-Madjlessi S, Surun P, Bentot C, Feteanu D, Lefebvre des Noettes V, et al. The cognitive disorders examination (Codex) is a reliable 3-minute test for detection of dementia in the elderly (validation study in 323 subjects). Presse Med. 2007a;36:1183-90.
4. Belmin J, Oasi C, Folio P, Pariel-Madjlessi S. Codex, un test ultra-rapide pour le repérage des démences chez les sujets âgés. Revue Geriatr. 2007b;32:627-31.
5. Borson S, Scanlan J, Brush M, Vitiliano P, Dokmak A. The Mini-Cog: a cognitive "vital signs" measure for dementia screening in multi-lingual elderly. Int J Geriatr Psychiatry. 2000;15:1021–7.
6. Brooke P, Bullock R. Validation of a 6 item cognitive impairment test with a view to primary care usage. Int J Geriatr Psychiatry. 1999;14:936–40.
7. Burns A, Lawlor B, Craig S. Assessment scales in old age psychiatry. 2nd ed. London: Martin Dunitz; 2004.
8. Cannon P, Larner AJ. Errors in the scoring and reporting of cognitive screening instruments administered in primary care. Neurodegener Dis Manag. 2016;6:271–6.
9. Chan CCH, Fage BA, Burton JK, Smailagic N, Gill SS, Herrmann N, et al. Mini-Cog for the diagnosis of Alzheimer's disease dementia and other dementias within a secondary care setting. Cochrane Database Syst Rev. 2019; 9:CD011414.
10. Connon P, Larner AJ. Six-item Cognitive Impairment Test (6CIT): diagnostic test accuracy study in primary care referrals. Int J Geriatr Psychiatry. 2017;32:583–4.

11. Fage BA, Chan CC, Gill SS, Noel-Storr AH. Herrmann N, Smailagic N, et al. Mini-Cog for the diagnosis of Alzheimer's disease dementia and other dementias within a community setting. Cochrane Database Syst Rev. 2015; 2:CD010860.
12. Gale TM, Larner AJ. Six-Item Cognitive Impairment Test (6CIT). In: Larner AJ, editor. Cognitive screening instruments. A practical approach. 2nd ed. London: Springer; 2017. p. 241–53.
13. Hodkinson HM. Evaluation of a mental test score for assessment of mental impairment in the elderly. Age Ageing. 1972;1:233–8.
14. Larner AJ. Codex (cognitive disorders examination) for the detection of dementia and mild cognitive impairment. Codex pour la détection de la démence et du mild cognitive impairment. Presse Med. 2013;42:e425–8.
15. Larner AJ. Implications of changing the Six-item Cognitive Impairment Test cutoff. Int J Geriatr Psychiatry. 2015;30:778–9.
16. Larner AJ, editor. Cognitive screening instruments. A practical approach. 2nd ed. London: Springer; 2017a.
17. Larner AJ. MMSE variants and subscores. In: Larner AJ (ed.). Cognitive screening instruments. A practical approach. 2nd ed. London: Springer; 2017b. p. 49–66.
18. Larner AJ. Mini-Mental State Examination: diagnostic test accuracy study in primary care referrals. Neurodegener Dis Manag. 2018;8:301–5.
19. Larner AJ. Evaluating cognitive screening instruments with the "likelihood to be diagnosed or misdiagnosed" measure. Int J Clin Pract. 2019a;73:e13265.
20. Larner AJ. New unitary metrics for dementia test accuracy studies. Prog Neurol Psychiatry. 2019b;23(3):21-5.
21. Larner AJ. Mini-Cog versus Codex (cognitive disorders examination): is there a difference? Dement Neuropsychol. 2020;accepted.
22. Mainland BJ, Shulman KI. Clock Drawing Test. In: Larner AJ, editor. Cognitive screening instruments. A practical approach. 2nd ed. London: Springer; 2017. p. 67–108.
23. Malmstrom TK, Voss VB, Cruz-Oliver DM, Cummings-Vaughn LA, Tumosa N, Grossberg GT, et al. The Rapid Cognitive Screen (RCS): a point-of-care screening for dementia and mild cognitive impairment. J Nutr Health Aging. 2015;19:741–4.
24. O'Caoimh R, Molloy DW. Comparing the diagnostic accuracy of two cognitive screening instruments in different dementia subtypes and clinical depression. Diagnostics (Basel). 2019;9:E93.
25. Piotrowicz K, Romanik W, Skalska A, et al. The comparison of the 1972 Hodkinson's Abbreviated Mental Test Score (AMTS) and its variants in screening for cognitive impairment. Aging Clin Exp Res. 2019;31:561–6.
26. Seitz DP, Chan CC, Newton HT, Gill SS, Herrmann N, Smailagic N, et al. Mini-Cog for the diagnosis of Alzheimer's disease dementia and other dementias within a primary care setting. Cochrane Database Syst Rev. 2018; 2:CD011415.
27. Vannier-Nitenberg C, Dauphinot V, Bongue B, Sass C, Bathsavanis A, Rouch I, et al. Performance of cognitive tests, individually and combined, for the detection of cognitive disorders amongst community-dwelling elderly people with memory complaints: the EVATEM study. Eur J Neurol. 2016;23:554–61.
28. Ziso B, Larner AJ. Codex (cognitive disorders examination) for the detection of dementia and mild cognitive impairment: diagnostic utility. J Neurol Neurosurg Psychiatry. 2013;84:e2.
29. Ziso B, Larner AJ. Codex (cognitive disorders examination) decision tree modified for the detection of dementia and MCI. Diagnostics (Basel). 2019;9:E58.

Chapter 5
Cognitive Screeners (2): Short Patient-Performance Scales (5–10 Min)

5.1 Introduction

Patient-performance scales are the most commonly applied cognitive screeners. A large range of tests is available (see, for example [5, 24]) which vary in length, item content, cognitive domains examined, and hence time to administer.

In this chapter pragmatic studies of patient-performance scales which ordinarily take between 5 and 10 minutes to administer are examined. These usually comprise around 10–20 items. A number of the screeners discussed here have been subjected to analysis using the new unitary metrics of LDM, SUI and NNSU [26, 27].

There are numerous other short patient-performance scales, at least one of which, the 7-minute screen [37], is explicit about its administration time,

Shorter and longer screening tests are considered elsewhere (Chaps. 4 and 6 respectively), as are informant scales (Chap. 7).

5.2 Mini-Mental State Examination (MMSE)

Origin:
Folstein MF, Folstein SE, McHugh PR. Mini-mental state. A practical method for grading the cognitive state of patients for the clinician. J Psychiatr Res. 1975;12:189–98 [10].
NB: Copyright Psychological Assessment Resources.

Content:
A 30-point cognitive screening instrument examining various cognitive domains, but heavily weighted toward language-related tasks. Memory and visuoperceptual testing is perfunctory and executive function testing is eschewed.

© Springer Nature Switzerland AG 2020
A. J. Larner, *Manual of Screeners for Dementia*,
https://doi.org/10.1007/978-3-030-41636-2_5

Orientation	10 (time 5, place 5)
Registration	3
Attention/Concentration (serial 7s or DLROW)	5 (best performed task)
Memory recall	3
Language naming	2
Language comprehension:	
"Close your eyes"	1
3 stage command	3
Language writing	1
Language repetition	1
Visuospatial abilities (intersecting pentagons)	1
Total score	**30**

Data:

Quantitative, discrete, ordinal. Score range 0–30, impaired to normal.

Pragmatic studies:

Larner AJ. Mini-Addenbrooke's Cognitive Examination: a pragmatic diagnostic accuracy study. Int J Geriatr Psychiatry. 2015a;30:547–8 [21].

Larner AJ. Mini-Addenbrooke's Cognitive Examination diagnostic accuracy for dementia: reproducibility study. Int J Geriatr Psychiatry. 2015b;30:1103–4 [22].

Results

(A) For diagnosis of dementia, cut-off <26/30 (from index study):

1. Demographics:

N	244
P = Prevalence of dementia (= pre-test probability)	0.18
Q = Level of the test	0.45

2. Paired measures of discrimination:

Sensitivity (Se), Specificity (Sp)	0.86, 0.64
PPV, NPV	0.34, 0.96
LR+, LR−	2.37 (moderate), 0.22 (moderate)
CUI+, CUI−	0.29 (very poor), 0.61 (adequate)

3. Unitary measures of discrimination:

Accuracy	0.68
Y	0.50
PSI	0.30
SUI	0.90 (poor)

4. Numbers needed:

To diagnose (NND)	2.00
To predict (NNP)	3.33
To misdiagnose (NNM)	3.13
Likelihood to be diagnosed or misdiagnosed (LDM = NNM/NND, NNM/NNP)	1.56, 0.94
For screening utility (NNSU)	1.11 (inadequate)

(B) For diagnosis of mild cognitive impairment, cut-off <26/30 (from index study):

1. Demographics:

N	201
P = Prevalence of mild cognitive impairment (= pre-test probability)	0.30
Q = Level of the test	0.36

2. Paired measures of discrimination:

Sensitivity (Se), Specificity (Sp)	0.67, 0.77
PPV, NPV	0.56, 0.84
LR+, LR−	2.94 (moderate), 0.43 (moderate)
CUI+, CUI−	0.38 (poor), 0.65 (good)

3. Unitary measures of discrimination:

Accuracy	0.74
Y	0.44
PSI	0.41
SUI	1.03 (adequate)

4. Numbers needed:

To diagnose (NND)	2.27
To predict (NNP)	2.44
To misdiagnose (NNM)	3.85
Likelihood to be diagnosed or misdiagnosed (LDM = NNM/NND, NNM/NNP)	1.69, 1.58
For screening utility (NNSU)	0.97 (adequate)

Conclusions:

In the more than 40 years since its original publication, MMSE has been very extensively used, although in recent years its fitness for purpose has been questioned [6] and its use superseded by newer screeners, a trend possibly exacerbated by the retrospective application of copyright. Nevertheless it still appears to be the most frequently used short screening test in many countries [12]. Generally MMSE has been found to have high specificity and low sensitivity for identification of dementia and mild cognitive impairment [34, 39, 40].

MMSE is relatively easy to administer and score in about 5–10 min. There may sometimes be issues around scoring, especially of the Attention/Concentration items.

Although sometimes characterised as an "interval scale" [16, p. 300–301], the differences between values at different points of the MMSE do not necessarily have the same meaning, hence in the nomenclature of Stevens [38] this is an ordinal rather than an interval scale. Similar considerations apply to other patient-performance and informant questionnaires examining cognitive function.

Data reported from these pragmatic studies, in which MMSE was compared with MACE (Sect. 5.4), showed better sensitivity than specificity. This reversal of the usual pattern of MMSE performance was also noted in a meta-analysis comparing it with ACE and ACE-R (Sects. 6.2 and 6.3; [31]). For diagnosis of both dementia and MCI, the LDM, SUI and NNSU metrics of MMSE were all ≈1.

In a previous publication [27] using data from another study of MMSE for MCI diagnosis [1], calculations showed higher NND (3.85) and NNP (3.85), lower NNM (3.03), and hence lower LDM values (both 0.79), than those reported here, despite using the same MMSE cut-off. Reasons for the discrepancy are not clear, but might possibly relate to disease prevalence (Sect. 14.3.1).

The combination of MMSE with other cognitive screening instruments (MoCA), informant scales (IQCODE, AD8), and functional scales (IADL Scale), has also been examined (Sects. 11.2, 11.3, 11.4, 12.4 respectively).

5.3   Mini-Mental Parkinson (MMP)

Origin:
Mahieux F, Michelet D, Manifacier M-J, Boller F, Fermanian J, Guillard A. Mini-Mental Parkinson: first validation study of a new bedside test constructed for Parkinson's disease. Behav Neurol. 1995;8:15–22 [32].

Content:
A 32-point cognitive screening instrument developed from the MMSE (Sect. 5.2) to detect cognitive impairment in patients with Parkinson's disease (PD). Orientation and attention items from the MMSE were retained, but in order to examine the visual and executive cognitive functions which are often impaired in PD the other MMSE items were substituted with tests of visual registration and recall, two set fluency, shifting, and concept processing.

Orientation	10 (as for MMSE)
Visual registration	3
Attention	5 (as for MMSE)
Two set fluency	3
Visual recall	4
Shifting	4
Concept processing	3
Total score	**32**

Data:
Quantitative, discrete, ordinal. Score range 0–32, impaired to normal.

Pragmatic studies: Larner AJ. Mini-Mental Parkinson (MMP) as a dementia screening test: comparison with the Mini-Mental State Examination (MMSE). Curr Aging Sci. 2012;5:136–9 [19].

Results
(A) For diagnosis of dementia, cut-off ≤17/32 (defined by optimal accuracy):

1. Demographics:

N	201
P = Prevalence of dementia (= pre-test probability)	0.23
Q = Level of the test	0.14

2. Paired measures of discrimination:

Sensitivity (Se), Specificity (Sp)	0.51, 0.97
PPV, NPV	0.83, 0.87
LR+, LR−	15.7 (very large), 0.51 (slight)
CUI+, CUI−	0.42 (poor), 0.84 (excellent)

3. Unitary measures of discrimination:

Accuracy	0.86
Y	0.48
PSI	0.70
SUI	1.26 (adequate)

4. Numbers needed:

To diagnose (NND)	2.08
To predict (NNP)	1.43
To misdiagnose (NNM)	7.14
Likelihood to be diagnosed or misdiagnosed (LDM = NNM/NND, NNM/NNP)	3.43, 5.00
For screening utility (NNSU)	0.79 (adequate)

(B) For diagnosis of mild cognitive impairment, cut-off ≤20/32 (defined by optimal accuracy):

1. Demographics:

N	154
P = Prevalence of mild cognitive impairment (= pre-test probability)	0.18
Q = Level of the test	0.12

2. Paired measures of discrimination:

Sensitivity (Se), Specificity (Sp)	0.29, 0.92
PPV, NPV	0.44, 0.85
LR+, LR−	3.59 (moderate), 0.78 (slight)
CUI+, CUI−	0.13 (very poor), 0.79 (good)

3. Unitary measures of discrimination:

Accuracy	0.81
Y	0.21
PSI	0.29
SUI	0.92 (poor)

1. Numbers needed:

To diagnose (NND)	4.76
To predict (NNP)	3.45
To misdiagnose (NNM)	5.26
Likelihood to be diagnosed or misdiagnosed (LDM = NNM/NND, NNM/NNP)	1.11, 1.53
For screening utility (NNSU)	1.09 (inadequate)

Conclusions:
MMP is relatively easy to administer and score in about 5–10 min. Materials other than pencil and paper are required for the visual registration and recall items.

This pragmatic study examined MMP as a general cognitive screening instrument, rather than exclusively for cognitive impairment in Parkinson's disease, hence broadening the potential applicability of the test. The rationale was that the changes in MMP addressed some of the shortcomings of neuropsychological coverage acknowledged to be present in MMSE. MMP has retained a place in cognitive assessment in PD [7].

Using the cut-offs defined by optimal test correct classification accuracy, the level of the test was low (Q=0.12, 0.14 for dementia and MCI respectively). MMP was found to be more specific than sensitive, as might have been anticipated from prior experience with MMSE, with good NPV, LR+, and CUI−. LDM, SUI and NNSU were all encouraging for dementia diagnosis, but not so for MCI, again as might have been anticipated from experience with MMSE.

Based on these data, MMP might be used as a general cognitive screening instrument for dementia diagnosis.

5.4 Mini-Addenbrooke's Cognitive Examination (MACE)

Origin:
Hsieh S, McGrory S, Leslie F, Dawson K, Ahmed S, Butler CR, et al. The Mini-Addenbrooke's Cognitive Examination: a new assessment tool for dementia. Dement Geriatr Cogn Disord. 2015;39:1–11 [11].

Content:

A 30-point cognitive screening instrument, a shortened version of the Addenbrooke's Cognitive Examination-Revised (ACE-R) and ACE-III (Sects. 6.3 and 6.4) developed by Mokken scaling analysis of these longer instruments.

Orientation (Time)	4
Registration (7-item name and address, Scored on third presentation)	7
Verbal fluency	7
Visuospatial abilities (Clock drawing)	5
Memory Recall	7
Total score	**30**

Data:

Quantitative, discrete, ordinal. Score range 0–30, impaired to normal.

Pragmatic studies:

Williamson J, Larner AJ. MACE for diagnosis of dementia and MCI: 3-year pragmatic diagnostic test accuracy study. Dement Geriatr Cogn Disord. 2018;45:300–7 [41].

Larner AJ. MACE for diagnosis of dementia and MCI: examining cut-offs and predictive values. Diagnostics (Basel). 2019c;9:E51 [28].

Results

(A) For diagnosis of dementia, cut-off $\leq$20/30 (defined by maximal Youden index):

1. Demographics:

N	755
P = Prevalence of dementia (= pre-test probability)	0.15
Q = Level of the test	0.39

2. Paired measures of discrimination:

Sensitivity (Se), Specificity (Sp)	0.91, 0.71
PPV, NPV	0.36, 0.98
LR+, LR−	3,11 (moderate), 0.12 (large)
CUI+, CUI−	0.33 (very poor), 0.70 (good)

3. Unitary measures of discrimination:

Accuracy	0.74
Y	0.62
PSI	0.34
SUI	1.03 (adequate)

4. Numbers needed:

To diagnose (NND)	1.61
To predict (NNP)	2.94
To misdiagnose (NNM)	3.85
Likelihood to be diagnosed or misdiagnosed (LDM = NNM/NND, NNM/NNP)	2.38, 1.31
For screening utility (NNSU)	0.97 (adequate)

(B) For diagnosis of mild cognitive impairment, cut-off ≤24/30 (defined by maximal Youden index):

1. Demographics:

N	641
P = Prevalence of mild cognitive impairment (= pre-test probability)	0.29
Q = Level of the test	0.59

2. Paired measures of discrimination:

Sensitivity (Se), Specificity (Sp)	0.90, 0.57
PPV, NPV	0.53, 0.92
LR+, LR−	2.11 (moderate), 0.17 (large)
CUI+, CUI−	0.48 (poor), 0.52 (adequate)

3. Unitary measures of discrimination:

Accuracy	0.69
Y	0.47
PSI	0.45
SUI	1.00 (adequate)

4. Numbers needed:

To diagnose (NND)	2.13
To predict (NNP)	2.22
To misdiagnose (NNM)	3.23
Likelihood to be diagnosed or misdiagnosed (LDM = NNM/NND, NNM/NNP)	1.52, 1.45
For screening utility (NNSU)	1.00 (adequate)

Conclusions:
MACE is a high sensitivity low specificity test with adequate unitary metrics for diagnosis of both dementia and MCI. Other metrics such as effect size (Cohen's d) also suggest MACE is a good brief screener for MCI [29, 30].

Compared to its parent screeners, ACE and ACE-R (Sects. 6.2 and 6.3), it appears to have retained sensitivity but sacrificed specificity, resulting in poorer LDM, SUI, and NNSU metrics, akin to those reported with MMSE and Free-Cog (Sects. 5.2 and 6.7 respectively).

5.5   Short Montreal Cognitive Assessment (s-MoCA)

Origin:
Roalf DR, Moore TM, Wolk DA, et al. Defining and validating a short form Montreal Cognitive Assessment (s-MoCA) for use in neurodegenerative disease. J Neurol Neurosurg Psychiatry. 2016;87:1303–10 [35].

Content:
A number of short-form versions of the Montreal Cognitive Assessment (MoCA; Sect. 6.5) have been described [33]. The one considered here is that developed by Roalf et al. [35] based on the 8 items of the MoCA found to be most discriminative by item response theory and computerised adaptive testing, producing a 16-point screening instrument.

Orientation	1 (Place)
Attention/Concentration (serial 7s)	3
Memory recall	5
Verbal fluency (lexical)	1
Language naming	1 (Rhinoceros)
Visuospatial abilities (Clock drawing)	3
Visuospatial abilities (Trail making)	1

Abstraction	1 (Measurement)
Total score	**16**

Data:
Quantitative, discrete, ordinal. Score range 0–16, impaired to normal.

Pragmatic studies:
Larner AJ. Short Montreal Cognitive Assessment: validation and reproducibility. J Geriatr Psychiatry Neurol. 2017b;30:104–8 [25].

Results
(A) For diagnosis of dementia, cut-off ≤12/16 (from index study):

1. Demographics:

N	260
P = Prevalence of dementia (= pre-test probability)	0.17
Q = Level of the test	0.74

2. Paired measures of discrimination:

Sensitivity (Se), Specificity (Sp)	0.98, 0.07
PPV, NPV	0.38, 0.83
LR+, LR−	1.05 (slight), 0.35 (moderate)
CUI+, CUI−	0.37 (poor), 0.06 (very poor)

3. Unitary measures of discrimination:

Accuracy	0.40
Y	0.05
PSI	0.21
SUI	0.43 (very poor)

4. Numbers needed:

To diagnose (NND)	20.0
To predict (NNP)	4.76
To misdiagnose (NNM)	1.67
Likelihood to be diagnosed or misdiagnosed (LDM = NNM/NND, NNM/NNP)	0.08, 0.35
For screening utility (NNSU)	2.33 (inadequate)

(B) For diagnosis of mild cognitive impairment, cut-off ≤12/16 (from index study):

1. Demographics:

N	217
P = Prevalence of mild cognitive impairment (= pre-test probability)	0.29
Q = Level of the test	0.69

2. Paired measures of discrimination:

Sensitivity (Se), Specificity (Sp)	0.93, 0.60
PPV, NPV	0.55, 0.94
LR+, LR−	2.33 (moderate), 0.11 (large)
CUI+, CUI−	0.51 (adequate), 0.56 (adequate)

3. Unitary measures of discrimination:

Accuracy	0.71
Y	0.53
PSI	0.49
SUI	1.07 (adequate)

4. Numbers needed:

To diagnose (NND)	1.89
To predict (NNP)	2.04
To misdiagnose (NNM)	3.45
Likelihood to be diagnosed or misdiagnosed (LDM = NNM/NND, NNM/NNP)	1.83, 1.69
For screening utility (NNSU)	0.93 (adequate)

Conclusions:

Studies of short forms of MoCA are in their infancy, although may be increasing [12]. The data from this pragmatic study of one particular s-MoCA form suggest it is a high sensitivity low specificity test with better metrics for identification of MCI, as might be anticipated from its origins, since the MoCA was specifically designed as a test to identify MCI (Sect. 6.5). Certainly LDM, SUI and NNSU values were more encouraging for MCI than for dementia.

5.6 DemTect

Origin:
Kalbe E, Calabrese P, Schwalen S, Kessler J. The Rapid Dementia Screening Test (RDST): a new economical tool for detecting possible patients with dementia. Dement Geriatr Cogn Disord. 2003;16:193–9 [13].
Kalbe E, Kessler J, Calabrese P, et al. DemTect: a new, sensitive cognitive screening test to support the diagnosis of mild cognitive impairment and early dementia. Int J Geriatr Psychiatry. 2004;19:136–43 [14].

Content:
A short screening test for dementia comprising five short subtests.

10 word list (×2)	3
Number transcoding	3
Semantic fluency	4
Reverse digit span	3
Delayed recall of word list	5
(Education ≤ 11 years +1)	
Total score	**18**

Data:
Quantitative, discrete, ordinal. Score range 0–18, impaired to normal, with correction for patient education, and with classification of final scores, as "suspected dementia" (≤8), "mild cognitive impairment" (9–12), and "appropriate for age" (13–18).

Pragmatic studies:
Larner AJ. DemTect in the diagnosis of dementia: first 100 patients. In: Iqbal K, Winblad B, Avila J, editors. Alzheimer's disease: new advances. Collection of selected articles of papers presented at the 10th International Conference on Alzheimer's disease and related disorders. Madrid, Spain, July 15–20, 2006. Bologna: Medimond; 2007a. p. 177–81 [17].
Larner AJ. DemTect: 1-year experience of a neuropsychological screening test for dementia. Age Ageing. 2007b;36:326–7 [18].

Results
For diagnosis of dementia, cut-off ≤8/18 (from index study):

1. Demographics:

N	111
P = Prevalence of cognitive impairment (= pre-test probability)	0.52
Q = Level of the test	0.58

2. Paired measures of discrimination:

Sensitivity (Se), Specificity (Sp)	0.84, 0.72
PPV, NPV	0.77, 0.81
LR+, LR−	2.99 (moderate), 0.22 (moderate)
CUI+, CUI−	0.65 (good), 0.58 (adequate)

3. Unitary measures of discrimination:

Accuracy	0.78
Y	0.56
PSI	0.58
SUI	1.23 (adequate)

4. Numbers needed:

To diagnose (NND)	1.79
To predict (NNP)	1.72
To misdiagnose (NNM)	4.55
Likelihood to be diagnosed or misdiagnosed (LDM = NNM/NND, NNM/NNP)	2.55, 2.64
For screening utility (NNSU)	0.81 (adequate)

Conclusions:
Despite its ease of use, correction to allow for patient educational level, and good metrics, with both high sensitivity and specificity for dementia diagnosis, DemTect does not seem to have achieved widespread use outside of Germanophone countries, despite the potentially helpful suggested classification of final scores [15]. In the pragmatic study LDM values were >2, and both SUI and NNSU were close to the threshold for a qualitative classification of good.

5.7 TYM-MCI (Hard-TYM)

Origin:
Brown J, Wiggins J, Dong H, Harvey R, Richardson F, Dawson K, Parker RA. The H-TYM. Evaluation of a short cognitive test to detect mild AD and amnestic MCI. Int J Geriatr Psychiatry. 2014;29:272–80 [2].
Brown JM, Lansdall CJ, Wiggins J, et al. The Test Your Memory for Mild Cognitive Impairment (TYM-MCI). J Neurol Neurosurg Psychiatry. 2017;88:1045–51 [3].

Content:

A more stringent version of Test Your Memory (TYM) test (Sect. 6.6) developed to detect mild AD and amnestic MCI by testing visual and verbal recall of recently learned material.

Data:

Quantitative, discrete, ordinal. Score range 0–30, impaired to normal. Subscores for verbal memory (0–15) and visual memory (0–15).

Pragmatic studies:

Larner AJ. Hard-TYM: a pragmatic study. Int J Geriatr Psychiatry. 2015c;30:330–1 [23].

Results

For diagnosis of mild cognitive impairment, cut-off ≤13/30 (from index study):

1. Demographics:

N	38
P = Prevalence of mild cognitive impairment (= pre-test probability)	0.16
Q = Level of the test	0.39

2. Paired measures of discrimination:

Sensitivity (Se), Specificity (Sp)	0.67, 0.66
PPV, NPV	0.27, 0.91
LR+, LR−	1.94 (slight), 0.51 (slight)
CUI+, CUI−	0.18 (very poor), 0.60 (adequate)

3. Unitary measures of discrimination:

Accuracy	0.66
Y	0.33
PSI	0.18
SUI	0.78 (poor)

4. Numbers needed:

To diagnose (NND)	3.03
To predict (NNP)	5.56

To misdiagnose (NNM)	2.94
Likelihood to be diagnosed or misdiagnosed (LDM = NNM/NND, NNM/NNP)	0.97, 0.53
For screening utility (NNSU)	1.28 (inadequate)

Conclusions:
Further studies of TYM-MCI, independent from the originators [4], are awaited. LDM, SUI, and NNSU metrics for MCI diagnosis from this pragmatic study were unimpressive but study numbers were small.

5.8   Frontal Assessment Battery (FAB)

Origin:
Dubois B, Slachevsky A, Litvan I, Pillon B. The FAB: a Frontal Assessment Battery at bedside. Neurology. 2000;55:1621–6 [9].

Content:
The Frontal Assessment Battery (FAB) identifies frontal lobe dysfunction, and hence differs from the general screeners discussed hitherto in this chapter. It may be useful in the identification of patients with the behavioural variant of fronto-temporal dementia (FTD).

Similarities (conceptualisation)	3
Lexical fluency (mental flexibility)	3
Motor series (programming)	3
Conflicting instructions (sensitivity to interference)	3
Go-No-Go (inhibitory control)	3
Prehension behaviour (environmental autonomy)	3
Total score	**18**

Data:
Quantitative, discrete, ordinal. Score range 0–18, impaired to normal.

Pragmatic studies:
Larner AJ. Can the Frontal Assessment Battery (FAB) help in the diagnosis of behavioural variant frontotemporal dementia? A pragmatic study. Int J Geriatr Psychiatry. 2013;28:106–7 [20].

Results
For diagnosis of bvFTD, cut-off ≤12/18 (from Slachevsky et al. [36]):

1. Demographics:

N	45
P = Prevalence of bvFTD (= pre-test probability)	0.36
Q = Level of the test	0.62

2. Paired measures of discrimination:

Sensitivity (Se), Specificity (Sp)	0.94, 0.55
PPV, NPV	0.54, 0.94
LR+, LR−	2.09 (moderate), 0.11 (large)
CUI+, CUI−	0.50 (adequate), 0.52 (adequate)

3. Unitary measures of discrimination:

Accuracy	0.69
Y	0.49
PSI	0.48
SUI	1.02 (adequate)

4. Numbers needed:

To diagnose (NND)	2.04
To predict (NNP)	2.08
To misdiagnose (NNM)	3.23
Likelihood to be diagnosed or misdiagnosed (LDM = NNM/NND, NNM/NNP)	1.58, 1.55
For screening utility (NNSU)	0.98 (adequate)

Conclusions:
FAB may be useful for bvFTD diagnosis on the basis of this small study but other reports have been less encouraging [8].

References

1. Abdel-Aziz K, Larner AJ. Six-item Cognitive Impairment Test (6CIT): pragmatic diagnostic accuracy study for dementia and MCI. Int Psychogeriatr. 2015;27:991–7.
2. Brown J, Wiggins J, Dong H, Harvey R, Richardson F, Dawson K, Parker RA. The H-TYM. Evaluation of a short cognitive test to detect mild AD and amnestic MCI. Int J Geriatr Psychiatry. 2014;29:272–80.

3. Brown JM, Lansdall CJ, Wiggins J, et al. The Test Your Memory for Mild Cognitive Impairment (TYM-MCI). J Neurol Neurosurg Psychiatry. 2017;88:1045–51.
4. Brown JM, Wiggins J, Dawson K, Rittman T, Rowe JB. Test Your Memory (TYM) and Test Your Memory for Mild Cognitive Impairment (TYM-MCI): a review and update including results of using the TYM Test in a general neurology clinic and using a telephone version of the TYM Test. Diagnostics (Basel). 2019;9:E116.
5. Burns A, Lawlor B, Craig S. Assessment scales in old age psychiatry. 2nd ed. London: Martin Dunitz; 2004.
6. Carnero-Pardo C. Should the Mini-Mental State Examination be retired? Neurologia. 2014;29:473–81.
7. Caslake R, Summers F, McConachie D, et al. The Mini-Mental Parkinson's (MMP) as a cognitive screening tool in people with Parkinson's disease. Curr Aging Sci. 2013;6:273–9.
8. Castiglioni S, Pelati O, Zuffi M, et al. The Frontal Assessment Battery does not differentiate frontotemporal dementia from Alzheimer's disease. Dement Geriatr Cogn Disord. 2006;22:125–31.
9. Dubois B, Slachevsky A, Litvan I, Pillon B. The FAB: a Frontal Assessment Battery at bedside. Neurology. 2000;55:1621–6.
10. Folstein MF, Folstein SE, McHugh PR. Mini-Mental State. A practical method for grading the cognitive state of patients for the clinician. J Psychiatr Res. 1975;12:189–98.
11. Hsieh S, McGrory S, Leslie F, Dawson K, Ahmed S, Butler CR, et al. The Mini-Addenbrooke's Cognitive Examination: a new assessment tool for dementia. Dement Geriatr Cogn Disord. 2015;39:1–11.
12. Judge D, Roberts J, Khandker RK, Ambegaonkar B, Black CM. Physician practice patterns associated with diagnostic evaluation of patients with suspected mild cognitive impairment and Alzheimer's disease. Int J Alzheimers Dis. 2019;2019:4942562.
13. Kalbe E, Calabrese P, Schwalen S, Kessler J. The Rapid Dementia Screening Test (RDST): a new economical tool for detecting possible patients with dementia. Dement Geriatr Cogn Disord. 2003;16:193–9.
14. Kalbe E, Kessler J, Calabrese P, et al. DemTect: a new, sensitive cognitive screening test to support the diagnosis of mild cognitive impairment and early dementia. Int J Geriatr Psychiatry. 2004;19:136–43.
15. Kalbe E, Kessler J. DemTect. In: Larner AJ (ed.). Cognitive screening instruments. A practical approach. 2nd ed. London: Springer; 2017. p. 197–208.
16. Kraemer HC, Taylor JL, Tinklenberg JR, Yesavage JA. The stages of Alzheimer's disease: a reappraisal. Dement Geriatr Cogn Disord. 1998;9:299–308.
17. Larner AJ. DemTect in the diagnosis of dementia: first 100 patients. In: Iqbal K, Winblad B, Avila J, editors. Alzheimer's disease: new advances. Collection of selected articles of papers presented at the 10th International Conference on Alzheimer's disease and related disorders. Madrid, Spain, July 15–20, 2006. Bologna: Medimond; 2007a:177–81.
18. Larner AJ. DemTect: 1-year experience of a neuropsychological screening test for dementia. Age Ageing. 2007b;36:326–7.
19. Larner AJ. Mini-Mental Parkinson (MMP) as a dementia screening test: comparison with the Mini-Mental State Examination (MMSE). Curr Aging Sci. 2012;5:136–9.
20. Larner AJ. Can the Frontal Assessment Battery (FAB) help in the diagnosis of behavioural variant frontotemporal dementia? A pragmatic study. Int J Geriatr Psychiatry. 2013;28:106–7.
21. Larner AJ. Mini-Addenbrooke's Cognitive Examination: a pragmatic diagnostic accuracy study. Int J Geriatr Psychiatry. 2015a;30:547–8.
22. Larner AJ. Mini-Addenbrooke's Cognitive Examination diagnostic accuracy for dementia: reproducibility study. Int J Geriatr Psychiatry. 2015b;30:1103–4.
23. Larner AJ. Hard-TYM: a pragmatic study. Int J Geriatr Psychiatry. 2015c;30:330–1.
24. Larner AJ, editor. Cognitive screening instruments. A practical approach. 2nd ed. London: Springer, 2017a.

25. Larner AJ. Short Montreal Cognitive Assessment: validation and reproducibility. J Geriatr Psychiatry Neurol. 2017b;30:104–8.
26. Larner AJ. Evaluating cognitive screening instruments with the "likelihood to be diagnosed or misdiagnosed" measure. Int J Clin Pract. 2019a;73:e13265.
27. Larner AJ. New unitary metrics for dementia test accuracy studies. Prog Neurol Psychiatry. 2019b;23(3):21–5.
28. Larner AJ. MACE for diagnosis of dementia and MCI: examining cut-offs and predictive values. Diagnostics (Basel). 2019c;9:E51.
29. Larner AJ. Diagnostic test accuracy studies in dementia. A pragmatic approach. 2nd ed. London: Springer; 2019d. p. 129.
30. Larner AJ. Free-Cog: pragmatic test accuracy study and comparison with Mini-Addenbrooke's Cognitive Examination (MACE). Dement Geriatr Cogn Disord. 2019e;47:254–63.
31. Larner AJ, Mitchell AJ. A meta-analysis of the accuracy of the Addenbrooke's Cognitive Examination (ACE) and the Addenbrooke's Cognitive Examination-Revised (ACE-R) in the detection of dementia. Int Psychogeriatr. 2014;26:555–63.
32. Mahieux F, Michelet D, Manifacier M-J, Boller F, Fermanian J, Guillard A. Mini-Mental Parkinson: first validation study of a new bedside test constructed for Parkinson's disease. Behav Neurol. 1995;8:15–22.
33. McDicken JA, Elliott E, Blayney G, Makin S, Ali M, Larner AJ, et al. Accuracy of the short-form Montreal Cognitive Assessment: systematic review and validation. Int J Geriatr Psychiatry. 2019;34:1515–25.
34. Mitchell AJ. The Mini-Mental State Examination (MMSE): update on its diagnostic accuracy and clinical utility for cognitive disorders. In: Larner AJ, editor. Cognitive screening instruments. A practical approach. 2nd ed. London: Springer; 2017. p. 37–48.
35. Roalf DR, Moore TM, Wolk DA, et al. Defining and validating a short form Montreal Cognitive Assessment (s-MoCA) for use in neurodegenerative disease. J Neurol Neurosurg Psychiatry. 2016;87:1303–10.
36. Slachevsky A, Villalpando JM, Sarazin M, Hahn BV, Pillon B, Dubois B. Frontal assessment battery and differential diagnosis of frontotemporal dementia and Alzheimer disease. Arch Neurol. 2004;61:1104–7.
37. Solomon PR, Hirschoff A, Kelly B, et al. A 7-minute neurocognitive screening battery highly sensitive to Alzheimer's disease. Arch Neurol. 1998;55:349–55.
38. Stevens SS. On the theory of scales of measurement. Science. 1946;103:677–80.
39. Tsoi KK, Chan JY, Hirai HW, Wong SY, Kwok TC. Cognitive tests to detect dementia. A systematic review and meta-analysis. JAMA Intern Med. 2015;175:1450–8.
40. Tsoi KK, Chan JY, Hirai HW, Wong A, Mok VC, Lam LC, et al. Recall tests are effective to detect mild cognitive impairment. A systematic review and meta-analysis of 108 diagnostic studies. J Am Med Dir Assoc. 2017;18:807.e17–29.
41. Williamson J, Larner AJ. MACE for diagnosis of dementia and MCI: 3-year pragmatic diagnostic test accuracy study. Dement Geriatr Cogn Disord. 2018;45:300–7.

Chapter 6
Cognitive Screeners (3): Longer Patient-Performance Scales (>10 min)

6.1 Introduction

In this chapter pragmatic studies of cognitive screeners which ordinarily take ≥ 10 min to administer are examined. Generally these comprise ≥ 20 items. There is some evidence that longer cognitive screeners may be more accurate, in terms of both correct classification accuracy and area under the receiver operating characteristic curve, than briefer cognitive screeners [18, 19]. A large range of tests is available (see, for example, [5, 21]).

Other cognitive instruments which may be too long for routine use in day-to-day clinical practice, such as the Alzheimer's Disease Assessment Scale-Cognitive Section (ADAS-Cog) and the Clinical Dementia Rating (CDR) scale, are not considered here, although they are often used as reference standards in research studies.

Shorter screening tests are considered elsewhere (Chaps. 4 and 5), as are informant scales (Chap. 7).

6.2 Addenbrooke's Cognitive Examination (ACE)

Origin:
Mathuranath PS, Nestor PJ, Berrios GE, Rakowicz W, Hodges JR. A brief cognitive test battery to differentiate Alzheimer's disease and frontotemporal dementia. Neurology. 2000;55:1613-20 [30].

Content:
A theoretically motivated cognitive screening test which attempted to address the neuropsychological omissions of the MMSE (which it incorporates) and to bridge the gap between very brief screening instruments and a full neuropsychological assessment for use in memory clinics.

Orientation	10 (time 5, place 5)
Registration	3
Attention/Concentration (serial 7 s or DLROW)	5 (best performed task)
Memory: recall	3
Memory: anterograde	28 (name and address)
Memory: retrograde	4
Verbal fluency	14 (lexical 7, semantic 7)
Language: naming	12
Language: comprehension	8
Language: repetition	5
Language: reading	2
Language: writing	1
Visuospatial abilities:	
Intersecting pentagons	1
Wire (Necker) cube	1
Clock drawing	3
Total score	**100**

Data:

Quantitative, discrete, ordinal. Score range 0–100, impaired to normal.

Pragmatic studies:

Larner AJ. Addenbrooke's Cognitive Examination (ACE) for the diagnosis and differential diagnosis of dementia. Clin Neurol Neurosurg. 2007;109:491–4 [14].

Results

For diagnosis of dementia, cut-off <75/100 (defined arbitrarily):

1. Demographics:

N	285
P = Prevalence of dementia (= pre-test probability)	0.49
Q = Level of the test	0.51

2. Paired measures of discrimination:

Sensitivity (Se), Specificity (Sp)	0.85, 0.83
PPV, NPV	0.83, 0.85
LR+, LR−	5.14 (large), 0.18 (large)
CUI+, CUI−	0.71 (good), 0.71 (good)

3. Unitary measures of discrimination:

Accuracy	0.84
Y	0.68
PSI	0.68
SUI	1.42 (good)

4. Numbers needed:

To diagnose (NND)	1.47
To predict (NNP)	1.47
To misdiagnose (NNM)	6.25
Likelihood to be diagnosed or misdiagnosed (LDM = NNM/NND, NNM/NNP)	4.25, 4.25
For screening utility (NNSU)	0.70 (good)

Conclusions:
The excellent metrics of the ACE have been confirmed in meta-analyses [28, 36]. The requirement to remove MMSE items from ACE because of copyright issues means that it is now superseded by ACE-III (Sect. 6.4; [10]). The excellent values of LDM, SUI, and NNSU in this pragmatic study are of note.

6.3 Addenbrooke's Cognitive Examination-Revised (ACE-R)

Origin:
Mioshi E, Dawson K, Mitchell J, Arnold R, Hodges JR. The Addenbrooke's Cognitive Examination Revised: a brief cognitive test battery for dementia screening. Int J Geriatr Psychiatry. 2006;21:1078–85 [32].

Content:
A development of the earlier ACE, also incorporating the MMSE, but with clearly defined subdomain scores.

Orientation	10 (time 5, place 5)
Registration	3
Attention/Concentration (serial 7 s or DLROW)	5 (best performed task)
Memory: recall	3

Memory: anterograde	19 (name and address)
Memory: retrograde	4
Verbal fluency	14 (lexical 7, semantic 7)
Language: naming	12
Language: comprehension	8
Language: repetition	4
Language: reading	1
Language: writing	1
Visuospatial abilities:	
Intersecting pentagons	1
Wire (Necker) cube	2
Clock drawing	5
Perceptual abilities:	
Dot counting	4
Fragmented letters	4
Total score	**100**

Data:
Quantitative, discrete, ordinal. Score range 0–100, impaired to normal.

Pragmatic studies:
Larner AJ. ACE-R: cross-sectional and longitudinal use for cognitive assessment. In: Fisher A, Hanin I (eds.). New trends in Alzheimer and Parkinson related disorders: ADPD 2009. Collection of selected free papers from the 9th International Conference on Alzheimer's and Parkinson's disease AD/PD. Prague, Czech Republic, March 11–15, 2009. Bologna: Medimond International Proceedings; 2009:103–7 [15].
Larner AJ. Addenbrooke's Cognitive Examination-Revised (ACE-R): pragmatic study of cross-sectional use for assessment of cognitive complaints of unknown aetiology. Int J Geriatr Psychiatry. 2013;28:547–8 [17].

Results
For diagnosis of dementia, cut-off ≤73/100 (defined by optimal accuracy):

1. Demographics:

N	243
P = Prevalence of dementia (= pre-test probability)	0.35
Q = Level of the test	0.37

2. Paired measures of discrimination:

Sensitivity (Se), Specificity (Sp)	0.87, 0.91
PPV, NPV	0.83, 0.93
LR+, LR−	9.21 (large), 0.14 (large)
CUI+, CUI−	0.72 (good), 0.85 (excellent)

3. Unitary measures of discrimination:

Accuracy	0.89
Y	0.78
PSI	0.76
SUI	1.57 (good)

4. Numbers needed:

To diagnose (NND)	1.28
To predict (NNP)	1.32
To misdiagnose (NNM)	9.09
Likelihood to be diagnosed or misdiagnosed (LDM = NNM/NND, NNM/NNP)	7.09, 6.91
For screening utility (NNSU)	0.64 (good)

Conclusions:
The excellent metrics of the ACE-R were confirmed in a separate pragmatic study based in an old age psychiatry clinic (dementia prevalence 0.51; [8]) and in meta-analyses [28, 36]. The requirement to remove MMSE items from ACE-R because of copyright issues means that it is now superseded by ACE-III (Sect. 6.4; [10]). The excellent values of LDM, SUI, and NNSU in this pragmatic study are of note.

The combination of ACE-R with an informant scale (IQCODE) and a functional scale (IADL Scale) has also been examined (Sects. 11.5 and 12.5 respectively).

6.4 ACE-III, ACEmobile

Origin:
Hsieh S, Schubert S, Hoon C, Mioshi E, Hodges JR. Validation of the Addenbrooke's Cognitive Examination III in frontotemporal dementia and Alzheimer's disease. Dement Geriatr Cogn Disord. 2013;36:242–50 [11].

Content:

A development of the earlier ACE and ACE-R but removing all the MMSE items to avoid copyright scores. ACE-III scores were highly correlated with ACE-R scores ($r = 0.99$).

Orientation	10 (time 5, place 5)
Registration	3
Attention/Concentration (serial 7 s only)	5
Memory: recall	3
Memory: anterograde	19 (name and address)
Memory: retrograde	4
Verbal fluency	14 (lexical 7, semantic 7)
Language: naming	12
Language: comprehension	7
Language: repetition	4
Language: reading	1
Language: writing	2
Visuospatial abilities:	
Intersecting lemnisci	1
Wire (Necker) cube	2
Clock drawing	5
Perceptual abilities:	
Dot counting	4
Fragmented letters	4
Total score	**100**

ACE-III is also available as an ipad based app, ACEmobile [34].

Data:

Quantitative, discrete, ordinal. Score range 0–100, impaired to normal.

Pragmatic studies:

None performed in this clinic, just occasional experience gained [24, 25, 29, 35, 38 Case 1].

Conclusions:

Results of pragmatic studies of ACE-III are likely to be similar to those recorded for ACE-R (Sect. 6.3), namely a high sensitivity and high specificity screener with good unitary (LDM, SUI, and NNSU) metrics.

A shorter version of ACE-III, the Mini- Addenbrooke's Cognitive Examination (MACE), has also been developed [12] (see Sect. 5.4).

6.5   Montreal Cognitive Assessment (MoCA)

Origin:
Nasreddine ZS, Phillips NA, Bédirian V, Charbonneau S, Whitehead V, Collin I, et al. The Montreal Cognitive Assessment, MoCA: a brief screening tool for mild cognitive impairment. J Am Geriatr Soc. 2005;53:695–9 [33].

Content:
MoCA was designed specifically to identify cases of Mild Cognitive Impairment, in contrast to the MMSE (Sect. 5.2) which was recognised to be insensitive to degrees of cognitive impairment insufficient to reach a diagnosis of dementia.

Orientation	6 (time 4, place 2)
Attention/Concentration	6 (serial 7 s: 3; repeating digits forwards or backwards: 2; tapping to sound of letter A: 1)
Memory: recall	5
Verbal fluency (lexical)	1
Language: naming	3
Language: repetition	2
Visuospatial abilities:	
Wire (Necker) cube	1
Clock drawing	3
Trail making	1
Abstraction	2
Total score	**30**

Data:
Quantitative, discrete, ordinal. Score range 0–30, impaired to normal.

Pragmatic studies:
Larner AJ. MACE versus MoCA: equivalence or superiority? Pragmatic diagnostic test accuracy study. Int Psychogeriatr. 2017b;29:931–7 [22].

Results
(A) For diagnosis of dementia, cut-off ≥26/30 (from index study):

1. Demographics:

N	260
P = Prevalence of dementia (= pre-test probability)	0.17
Q = Level of the test	0.74

2. Paired measures of discrimination:

Sensitivity (Se), Specificity (Sp)	1.00, 0.31
PPV, NPV	0.22, 1.00
LR+, LR−	1.46 (slight), ∝ (very large)
CUI+, CUI−	0.22 (very poor), 0.31 (very poor)

3. Unitary measures of discrimination:

Accuracy	0.43
Y	0.31
PSI	0.22
SUI	0.53 (very poor)

4. Numbers needed:

To diagnose (NND)	3.23
To predict (NNP)	4.55
To misdiagnose (NNM)	1.75
Likelihood to be diagnosed or misdiagnosed (LDM = NNM/NND, NNM/NNP)	0.54, 0.39
For screening utility (NNSU)	1.89 (inadequate)

(B) For diagnosis of mild cognitive impairment, cut-off ≥26/30 (from index study):

1. Demographics:

N	217
P = Prevalence of mild cognitive impairment (= pre-test probability)	0.35
Q = Level of the test	0.69

2. Paired measures of discrimination:

Sensitivity (Se), Specificity (Sp)	0.92, 0.44
PPV, NPV	0.46, 0.91
LR+, LR−	1.63 (slight), 0.18 (large)
CUI+, CUI−	0.43 (poor), 0.40 (poor)

3. Unitary measures of discrimination:

Accuracy	0.60
Y	0.36
PSI	0.37
SUI	0.83 (poor)

4. Numbers needed:

To diagnose (NND)	2.78
To predict (NNP)	2.70
To misdiagnose (NNM)	2.50
Likelihood to be diagnosed or misdiagnosed (LDM = NNM/NND, NNM/NNP)	0.90, 0.93
For screening utility (NNSU)	1.20 (inadequate)

Conclusions:
The MoCA has become very widely used since its original description for the assessment of many cognitive disorders [13].

The results of this pragmatic study confirm those of a previous study in the same clinic [16, 20, 23], namely that MoCA is a high sensitivity, low specificity test. However, meta-analyses have found both high sensitivity and specificity for diagnosis of both dementia and MCI [6, 7, 36, 37] and certainly LDM values were much improved when examining meta-analytic data [39] in comparison to this pragmatic study, which also had poor SUI and inadequate NNSU.

Short versions of the MoCA have also been developed [31] (see Sect. 5.5).

6.6   Test Your Memory (TYM) Test

Origin:
Brown J, Pengas G, Dawson K, Brown LA, Clatworthy P. Self administered cognitive screening test (TYM) for detection of Alzheimer's disease: cross sectional study. BMJ. 2009;338:b2030 [2].

Content:
The Test Your Memory (TYM) test is a 10-item cognitive test instrument which is self-administered under medical supervision.

Orientation	10
Copying	2
Retrograde memory	3
Calculation	4
Fluency (phonemic)	4
Similarities	4
Naming	5
Visuospatial 1 and 2 (clock)	7
Anterograde memory	6
Executive	5
Total score	**50**

Data:

Quantitative, discrete, ordinal. Score range 0–50, impaired to normal.

Pragmatic studies:

Hancock P, Larner AJ. Test Your Memory (TYM) test: diagnostic utility in a memory clinic population. Int J Geriatr Psychiatry. 2011;26:976–80 [9].

Larner AJ. Short performance-based cognitive screening instruments for the diagnosis of mild cognitive impairment. Prog Neurol Psychiatry. 2016;20(2):21–6 [20].

Results

(A) For diagnosis of dementia, cut-off ≤30/50 (defined by optimal accuracy):

1. Demographics:

N	224
P = Prevalence of dementia (= pre-test probability)	0.35
Q = Level of the test	0.33

2. Paired measures of discrimination:

Sensitivity (Se), Specificity (Sp)	0.73, 0.88
PPV, NPV	0.77, 0.86
LR+, LR−	6.28 (large), 0.30 (moderate)
CUI+, CUI−	0.56 (adequate), 0.76 (good)

3. Unitary measures of discrimination:

Accuracy	0.83
Y	0.61

| PSI | 0.63 |
| SUI | 1.32 (good) |

4. Numbers needed:

To diagnose (NND)	1.64
To predict (NNP)	1.59
To misdiagnose (NNM)	5.88
Likelihood to be diagnosed or misdiagnosed (LDM = NNM/NND, NNM/NNP)	3.59, 3.71
For screening utility (NNSU)	0.76 (good)

(B) For diagnosis of mild cognitive impairment, cut-off ≤42/50 (from index study):

1. Demographics:

N	146
P = Prevalence of mild cognitive impairment (= pre-test probability)	0.27
Q = Level of the test	0.55

2. Paired measures of discrimination:

Sensitivity (Se), Specificity (Sp)	0.79, 0.54
PPV, NPV	0.39, 0.88
LR+, LR−	1.74 (slight), 0.38 (moderate)
CUI+, CUI−	0.31 (very poor), 0.48 (poor)

3. Unitary measures of discrimination:

Accuracy	0.61
Y	0.33
PSI	0.27
SUI	0.79 (poor)

4. Numbers needed:

| To diagnose (NND) | 3.03 |
| To predict (NNP) | 3.70 |

To misdiagnose (NNM)	2.56
Likelihood to be diagnosed or misdiagnosed (LDM = NNM/NND, NNM/NNP)	0.85, 0.69
For screening utility (NNSU)	1.27 (inadequate)

Conclusions:
As a patient self-administered test, TYM has potential advantages in situations where clinician time is limited, and certainly the test has achieved a reasonable degree of uptake [1, 3]. However, the qualitative aspect of cognitive screening in the patient-clinician interaction is lost, and there may be an increased chance of patient dropout from test completion unless supervised by other staff. LDM, SUI, and NNSU metrics for dementia diagnosis look encouraging in the pragmatic study, but less so for MCI.

Initially evaluated for the detection of Alzheimer's disease, TYM may also be used in the evaluation of non-Alzheimer dementias, as well as proving useful in general neurology clinics and as a telephone-administered test [3, 4].

6.7   Free-Cog

Origin:
Burns, A. Personal communication, 2017.

Content:
A 30-point cognitive screening instrument incorporating assessment of both cognition and function.

Cognitive function:	
General knowledge	1
Orientation	6 (Time 3, Place 3)
Calculation	3
Attention/Concentration (serial 7 s or DLROW)	2
Memory recall (5 words, previously presented)	5
Verbal fluency (semantic: animals)	1
Language naming	2
Language writing	1
Language repetition	1
Visuospatial abilities (Clock drawing)	3

Cognitive function:	
Executive function:	
Five questions relating to: social function, travel, home, emergency, and self-care function	5
Total score	**30**

Data:

Quantitative, discrete, ordinal. Score range 0–30, impaired to normal. Subscores for cognitive function (0–25) and executive function (0–5).

Pragmatic studies:

Larner AJ. Free-Cog: pragmatic test accuracy study and comparison with Mini-Addenbrooke's Cognitive Examination. Dement Geriatr Cogn Disord. 2019c;47:254–63 [26].

Results

(A) For diagnosis of dementia, cut-off ≤22/30 (defined by maximal Youden index):

1. Demographics:

N	141
P = Prevalence of dementia (= pre-test probability)	0.11
Q = Level of the test	0.40

2. Paired measures of discrimination:

Sensitivity (Se), Specificity (Sp)	1.00, 0.67
PPV, NPV	0.27, 1.00
LR+, LR−	3.07 (moderate), 0 (very large)
CUI+, CUI-	0.27 (very poor), 0.67 (good)

3. Unitary measures of discrimination:

Accuracy	0.71
Y	0.67
PSI	0.27
SUI	0.94 (poor)

4. Numbers needed:

To diagnose (NND)	1.49
To predict (NNP)	3.70
To misdiagnose (NNM)	3.45
Likelihood to be diagnosed or misdiagnosed (LDM = NNM/NND, NNM/NNP)	2.31, 0.93
For screening utility (NNSU)	1.06 (inadequate)

(B) For diagnosis of mild cognitive impairment, cut-off ≤22/30 (defined by maximal Youden index):

1. Demographics:

N	126
P = Prevalence of mild cognitive impairment (= pre-test probability)	0.32
Q = Level of the test	0.33

2. Paired measures of discrimination:

Sensitivity (Se), Specificity (Sp)	0.58, 0.81
PPV, NPV	0.63, 0.78
LR+, LR−	3.12 (moderate), 0.52 (slight)
CUI+, CUI−	0.37 (poor), 0.63 (adequate)

3. Unitary measures of discrimination:

Accuracy	0.73
Y	0.39
PSI	0.41
SUI	1.00 (good)

4. Numbers needed:

To diagnose (NND)	2.56
To predict (NNP)	2.44
To misdiagnose (NNM)	3.70
Likelihood to be diagnosed or misdiagnosed (LDM = NNM/NND, NNM/NNP)	1.44, 1.52
For screening utility (NNSU)	1.00 (adequate)

Conclusions:

The results from this pragmatic study are comparable in terms of LDM, SUI and NNSU to those reported for MMSE (Sect. 5.2). The study suggested Free-Cog may be used as a screening assessment for dementia in dedicated cognitive disorders clinics but for MCI screening its performance is less suitable, and probably inferior to MACE (Sect. 5.4). Free-Cog has also been used in individual cases [27].

References

1. Brown JM. TYM (Test Your Memory) testing. In: Larner AJ, editor. Cognitive screening instruments. A practical approach, 2nd ed. London: Springer; 2017. p. 209–29.
2. Brown J, Pengas G, Dawson K, Brown LA, Clatworthy P. Self administered cognitive screening test (TYM) for detection of Alzheimer's disease: cross sectional study. BMJ. 2009;338:b2030.
3. Brown JM, Wiggins J, Dawson K, Rittman T, Rowe JB. Test Your Memory (TYM) and Test Your Memory for Mild Cognitive Impairment (TYM-MCI): a review and update including results of using the TYM Test in a general neurology clinic and using a telephone version of the TYM Test. Diagnostics. 2019a;9:E116.
4. Brown JM, Wiggins J, Lansdall CJ, Dawson K, Rittman T, Rowe JB. Test Your Memory (TYM test): diagnostic evaluation of patients with non-Alzheimer dementias. J Neurol. 2019b;266:2546–53.
5. Burns A, Lawlor B, Craig S. Assessment scales in old age psychiatry. 2nd ed. London: Martin Dunitz; 2004.
6. Ciesielska N, Sokolowski R, Mazue E, Podhorecka M, Polak-Szabela A, Kedziora-Kornatowska K. Is the Montreal Cognitive Assessment (MoCA) test better suited than the Mini-Mental State Examination (MMSE) in mild cognitive impairment (MCI) detection among people aged over 60? Meta-analysis. Psychiatr Pol. 2016;50:1039–52.
7. Davis DH, Creavin ST, Yip JL, Noel-Storr AH, Brayne C, Cullum S. Montreal Cognitive Assessment for the diagnosis of Alzheimer's disease and other dementias. Cochrane Database Syst Rev. 2015;10:CD010775.
8. Hancock P, Larner AJ. Diagnostic utility of the Informant Questionnaire on Cognitive Decline in the Elderly (IQCODE) and its combination with the Addenbrooke's Cognitive Examination-Revised (ACE-R) in a memory clinic-based population. Int Psychogeriatr. 2009;21:526–30.
9. Hancock P, Larner AJ. Test Your Memory (TYM) test: diagnostic utility in a memory clinic population. Int J Geriatr Psychiatry. 2011;26:976–80.
10. Hodges JR, Larner AJ. Addenbrooke's Cognitive Examinations: ACE, ACE-R, ACE-III, ACEapp, and M-ACE. In: Larner AJ (ed.). Cognitive screening instruments. A practical approach, 2nd ed. London: Springer; 2017. p. 109–37.
11. Hsieh S, Schubert S, Hoon C, Mioshi E, Hodges JR. Validation of the Addenbrooke's Cognitive Examination III in frontotemporal dementia and Alzheimer's disease. Dement Geriatr Cogn Disord. 2013;36:242-50.
12. Hsieh S, McGrory S, Leslie F, Dawson K, Ahmed S, Butler CR, et al. The Mini-Addenbrooke's Cognitive Examination: a new assessment tool for dementia. Dement Geriatr Cogn Disord. 2015;39:1–11.
13. Julayanont P, Nasreddine ZS. Montreal Cognitive Assessment (MoCA): concept and clinical review. In: Larner AJ, editor. Cognitive screening instruments. A practical approach, 2nd ed. London: Springer; 2017. p. 139–95.
14. Larner AJ. Addenbrooke's Cognitive Examination (ACE) for the diagnosis and differential diagnosis of dementia. Clin Neurol Neurosurg. 2007;109:491–4.
15. Larner AJ. ACE-R: cross-sectional and longitudinal use for cognitive assessment. In: Fisher A, Hanin I, editors. New trends in Alzheimer and Parkinson related disorders: ADPD 2009.

Collection of selected free papers from the 9th International Conference on Alzheimer's and Parkinson's disease AD/PD. Prague, Czech Republic, p. 11–15, 2009. Bologna: Medimond International Proceedings; 2009:103–7.

16. Larner AJ. Screening utility of the Montreal Cognitive Assessment (MoCA): in place of—or as well as—the MMSE? Int Psychogeriatr. 2012;24:391–6.

17. Larner AJ. Addenbrooke's Cognitive Examination-Revised (ACE-R): pragmatic study of cross-sectional use for assessment of cognitive complaints of unknown aetiology. Int J Geriatr Psychiatry. 2013;28:547–8.

18. Larner AJ. Speed versus accuracy in cognitive assessment when using CSIs. Prog Neurol Psychiatry. 2015a;19(1):21–4.

19. Larner AJ. Performance-based cognitive screening instruments: an extended analysis of the time versus accuracy trade-off. Diagnostics (Basel). 2015b;5:504–12.

20. Larner AJ. Short performance-based cognitive screening instruments for the diagnosis of mild cognitive impairment. Prog Neurol Psychiatry. 2016;20(2):21–6.

21. Larner AJ, editor. Cognitive screening instruments. A practical approach, 2nd edition. London: Springer;2017a.

22. Larner AJ. MACE versus MoCA: equivalence or superiority? Pragmatic diagnostic test accuracy study. Int Psychogeriatr. 2017b;29:931–7.

23. Larner AJ. Short Montreal Cognitive Assessment: validation and reproducibility. J Geriatr Psychiatry Neurol. 2017c;30:104–8.

24. Larner AJ. Dual pathology or unifying diagnosis? J R Coll Physicians Edinb. 2019a;49:145–6.

25. Larner AJ. *Scrabble*-ing with dementia. Adv Clin Neurosci Rehabil. 2019b;18(4):25.

26. Larner AJ. Free-Cog: pragmatic test accuracy study and comparison with Mini-Addenbrooke's Cognitive Examination. Dement Geriatr Cogn Disord. 2019c;47:254–63.

27. Larner AJ. Spontaneous resolution of frontotemporal brain sagging syndrome. Clin Med. 2019d;19:428.

28. Larner AJ, Mitchell AJ. A meta-analysis of the accuracy of the Addenbrooke's Cognitive Examination (ACE) and the Addenbrooke's Cognitive Examination-Revised (ACE-R) in the detection of dementia. Int Psychogeriatr. 2014;26:555–63.

29. Lees RA, Hendry K, Broomfield N, Stott D, Larner AJ, Quinn TJ. Cognitive assessment in stroke: feasibility and test properties using differing approaches to scoring of incomplete items. Int J Geriatr Psychiatry. 2017;32:1072–8.

30. Mathuranath PS, Nestor PJ, Berrios GE, Rakowicz W, Hodges JR. A brief cognitive test battery to differentiate Alzheimer's disease and frontotemporal dementia. Neurology. 2000;55:1613–20.

31. McDicken JA, Elliott E, Blayney G, Makin S, Ali M, Larner AJ, et al. Accuracy of the short-form Montreal Cognitive Assessment: systematic review and validation. Int J Geriatr Psychiatry. 2019;34:1515–25.

32. Mioshi E, Dawson K, Mitchell J, Arnold R, Hodges JR. The Addenbrooke's Cognitive Examination Revised: a brief cognitive test battery for dementia screening. Int J Geriatr Psychiatry. 2006;21:1078–85.

33. Nasreddine ZS, Phillips NA, Bédirian V, Charbonneau S, Whitehead V, Collin I, et al. The Montreal Cognitive Assessment, MoCA: a brief screening tool for mild cognitive impairment. J Am Geriatr Soc. 2005;53:695–9.

34. Newman CGJ, Bevins AD, Zajicek JP, et al. Improving the quality of cognitive screening assessments: ACEmobile, an iPad-based version of the Addenbrooke's Cognitive Examination-III. Alzheimers Dement. 2017;10:182–7.

35. St John L, Larner AJ. Muscle wasting, bone pain and cognitive decline: a unifying diagnosis. Br J Hosp Med. 2015;76:602–3.

36. Tsoi KK, Chan JY, Hirai HW, Wong SY, Kwok TC. Cognitive tests to detect dementia. A systematic review and meta-analysis. JAMA Intern Med. 2015;175: 1450–8.

37. Tsoi KK, Chan JY, Hirai HW, Wong A, Mok VC, Lam LC, et al. Recall tests are effective to detect mild cognitive impairment. A systematic review and meta-analysis of 108 diagnostic studies. J Am Med Dir Assoc. 2017;18:807.e17–29.

38. Williamson JC, Bonello M, Larner AJ. Genetic investigation in dementia: new interpretive challenges. Prog Neurol Psychiatry. 2018;22(4):6–8.

39. Williamson JC, Larner AJ. "Likelihood to be diagnosed or misdiagnosed": application to meta-analytic data for cognitive screening instruments. Neurodegener Dis Manag. 2019;9:91–5.

Chapter 7
Cognitive Screeners (4): Informant Scales

7.1 Introduction

Obtaining collateral information is a key aspect of cognitive assessment, usually by interviewing a knowledgeable informant (spouse, child, carer). Use of collateral history from an informant (heteroamnesis) is recommended in many clinical diagnostic criteria and guidelines for dementia. This informant input to the screening process may be formalised by administration of validated informant scales.

Since many people attend the cognitive clinic alone despite a written request to attend with a knowledgeable informant (the "attended alone" sign, Sect. 3.2), the case mix in studies of informant scales is different from that in which patient-performance scales are examined, with a higher prevalence of cognitively impaired individuals, since most patients who attend alone do not have cognitive impairment.

Some functional scales (see Chap. 9) might also have been included here, since for their completion informant input may be mandatory (e.g. Zarit Burden Interview, ZBI; Sect. 9.3) or optional (e.g. Instrumental Activities of Daily Living (IADL) Scale; Sect. 9.2). Informant report is also required in Cornell Scale for Depression in Dementia (Sect. 8.4).

A number of instruments which combine informant report with patient report or patient performance have been described such as the General Practitioner Assessment of Cognition (GPCOG [4, 23]), BrainCheck [8], Cognitive Function Instrument (CFI [2]), and the Brief Assessment of Impaired Cognition (BASIC [16]). Combining some individual patient and informant screeners is examined in Chap. 11.

© Springer Nature Switzerland AG 2020   89
A. J. Larner, *Manual of Screeners for Dementia*,
https://doi.org/10.1007/978-3-030-41636-2_7

7.2   Ascertain Dementia-8 (AD8)

Origin:
Galvin JE, Roe CM, Powlishta KK, et al. The AD8. A brief informant interview to detect dementia. Neurology. 2005;65:559–64 [10].

Content:
AD8, or Ascertain Dementia-8, is a brief informant screening questionnaire for dementia. Each of a series of 8 statements is graded by the informant as yes, no, or don't know, the overall score being given by the sum of "yes" responses (range 0–8), with the specified cut-offs being:

- 0–1: normal cognition
- 2 or greater: cognitive impairment is likely to be present.

Data:
Quantitative, discrete, ordinal. Score range 8–0, impaired to normal (i.e. negatively scored). AD8 therefore correlates negatively with most cognitive screening instruments which are scored positively.

Pragmatic studies:
Larner AJ. AD8 informant questionnaire for cognitive impairment: pragmatic diagnostic test accuracy study. J Geriatr Psychiatry Neurol. 2015;28:198–202 [19].

Connon P, Larner A. Combining informant (AD8) and patient (MACE) cognitive screening. J Neurol Neurosurg Psychiatry. 2017;88(Suppl1):A20 (PO030) [7].

Results
(A) For diagnosis of dementia, cut-off ≥2/8:

1. Demographics:

N	279
P = Prevalence of dementia (= pre-test probability)	0.30
Q = Level of the test	0.92

2. Paired measures of discrimination:

Sensitivity (Se), Specificity (Sp)	0.98, 0.10
PPV, NPV	0.32, 0.91
LR+, LR−	1.09 (slight), 0.24 (moderate)
CUI+, CUI−	0.31 (very poor), 0.09 (very poor)

3. Unitary measures of discrimination:

Accuracy	0.36
Y	0.08
PSI	0.23
SUI	0.40 (very poor)

4. Numbers needed:

To diagnose (NND)	12.8
To predict (NNP)	4.46
To misdiagnose (NNM)	1.57
Likelihood to be diagnosed or misdiagnosed (LDM = NNM/NND, NNM/NNP)	0.12, 0.35
For screening utility (NNSU)	2.50 (inadequate)

(B) For diagnosis of mild cognitive impairment, cut-off $\geq 2/8$:

1. Demographics:

N	196
P = Prevalence of mild cognitive impairment (= pre-test probability)	0.48
Q = Level of the test	0.90

2. Paired measures of discrimination:

Sensitivity (Se), Specificity (Sp)	0.97, 0.17
PPV, NPV	0.52, 0.85
LR+, LR−	5.81 (large), 0.19 (large)
CUI+, CUI−	0.50 (adequate), 0.14 (very poor)

3. Unitary measures of discrimination:

Accuracy	0.55
Y	0.14
PSI	0.37
SUI	0.64 (very poor)

4. Numbers needed:

To diagnose (NND)	7.14
To predict (NNP)	2.70
To misdiagnose (NNM)	2.23
Likelihood to be diagnosed or misdiagnosed (LDM = NNM/NND, NNM/NNP)	0.31, 0.82
For screening utility (NNSU)	1.56 (inadequate)

Conclusions:

AD8 was found to be very sensitive but not specific in the studies in the author's clinic. The latter finding was not corroborated by other studies of AD8 included in reviews and meta-analyses [5, 9, 15]. Hence the poor LDM metrics in the clinic studies (all <1) differed from those in the meta-analyses (all >1; [28]). This may relate to the case mix encountered in the particular study settings. SUI and NNSU values were also suboptimal in the individual studies, both parameters failing to achieve "adequate" classification.

AD8 has also been administered in a dedicated epilepsy clinic where a high frequency of cognitive impairment was found in patients with epilepsy in both self-rating and informant assessments [1].

The combination of AD8 with cognitive screening instruments (MMSE, 6CIT, MoCA, MACE) has also been examined (Sects. 11.4, 11.6, 11.7, and 11.8 respectively).

7.3   Informant Questionnaire on Cognitive Decline in the Elderly (IQCODE)

Origin:

Jorm AF, Jacomb PA. The Informant Questionnaire on Cognitive Decline in the Elderly (IQCODE): socio-demographic correlates, reliability, validity and some norms. Psychol Med. 1989;19:1015–22 [17].

Content:

The Informant Questionnaire on Cognitive Decline in the Elderly (IQCODE) in its original formulation asks an informant about change in a person's everyday cognitive function over a 10-year period through a series of 26 statements which are graded by the informant on a five point scale:

- 1: much improved
- 2: a bit improved

- 3: not much change
- 4: a bit worse
- 5: much worse.

The overall score is given by the sum of these responses divided by the total number of responses given; up to three missing items are generally permitted. Shorter forms of IQCODE (16- or 7-item) or covering a shorter time frame (2 years as opposed to 10 years) have also been reported.

Data:

Quantitative, discrete, ordinal. Score range = 1–5, higher scores suggest greater impairment. IQCODE correlates negatively with most cognitive screening instruments.

Pragmatic studies:

Hancock P, Larner AJ. Diagnostic utility of the Informant Questionnaire on Cognitive Decline in the Elderly (IQCODE) and its combination with the Addenbrooke's Cognitive Examination-Revised (ACE-R) in a memory clinic-based population. Int Psychogeriatr. 2009;21:526–30 [12].

Results
For diagnosis of dementia, cut-off ≥3.6/5:

1. Demographics:

N	144
P = Prevalence of dementia (= pre-test probability)	0.59
Q = Level of the test	0.76

2. Paired measures of discrimination:

Sensitivity (Se), Specificity (Sp)	0.86, 0.39
PPV, NPV	0.67, 0.66
LR+, LR−	1.41 (slight), 0.36 (moderate)
CUI+, CUI−	0.58 (adequate), 0.26 (very poor)

3. Unitary measures of discrimination:

Accuracy	0.67
Y	0.25
PSI	0.33
SUI	0.84 (poor)

4. Numbers needed:

To diagnose (NND)	4.00
To predict (NNP)	3.03
To misdiagnose (NNM)	3.03
Likelihood to be diagnosed or misdiagnosed (NNM/NND, NNM/NNP)	0.76, 1.00
For screening utility (NNSU)	1.19 (inadequate)

Conclusions:
IQCODE has become widely applied for the assessment of cognitive function [6, 13, 14, 22]. Although LDM values for IQCODE in the pragmatic study were suboptimal (≤ 1), as were SUI and NNSU, both parameters failing to achieve "adequate" classification, an analysis of data from meta-analyses [21, 24] showed better LDMs (>2, >3, respectively; [27]).

The combination of IQCODE with cognitive screening instruments (MMSE, ACE-R) has also been examined (Sects. 11.3 and 11.5 respectively).

7.4 Cambridge Behavioural Inventory (CBI)

Origin:
Wedderburn C, Wear H, Brown J, et al. The utility of the Cambridge Behavioural Inventory in neurodegenerative disease. J Neurol Neurosurg Psychiatry. 2008;79:500–3 [26].

Content:
Short, self-administered, informant questionnaire with 81 items in 13 subsections.

Memory	6 items
Orientation and attention	7 items
Everyday skills	8 items
Self-care	7 items
Mood	9 items
Beliefs	7 items
Challenging behaviour	4 items
Disinhibition	5 items
Eating habits	5 items
Sleep	2 items
Stereotypic and motor behaviours	11 items

Motivation	8 items
Insight/awareness	2 items
Total score	**81 items**

Informants are asked to score the various behavioural and psychiatric symptoms subjectively according to a frequency-based intensity scale (for most symptoms minimum = 0, not present; maximum = 4, constantly present).

Data:
Quantitative, discrete, ordinal. Possible score range of global CBI = 0–324 (normal to impaired).

Pragmatic studies:
Hancock P, Larner AJ. Cambridge Behavioural Inventory for the diagnosis of dementia. Prog Neurol Psychiatry. 2008;12(7):23–5 [11].

Larner AJ. Dementia in clinical practice: a neurological perspective. Pragmatic studies in the Cognitive Function Clinic. 3rd edition. London: Springer; 2018: 142–5 [20].

Results
For diagnosis of dementia, cut-off >80/324:

1. Demographics:

N	159
P = Prevalence of dementia (= pre-test probability)	0.63
Q = Level of the test	0.43

2. Paired measures of discrimination:

Sensitivity (Se), Specificity (Sp)	0.54, 0.75
PPV, NPV	0.78, 0.49
LR+, LR−	2.12 (moderate), 0.62 (slight)
CUI+, CUI−	0.42 (poor), 0.37 (poor)

3. Unitary measures of discrimination:

Accuracy	0.62
Y	0.29
PSI	0.27
SUI	0.79 (poor)

4. Numbers needed:

To diagnose (NND)	3.45
To predict (NNP)	3.70
To misdiagnose (NNM)	2.63
Likelihood to be diagnosed or misdiagnosed (LDM = NNM/NND, NNM/NNP)	0.76, 0.71
For screening utility (NNSU)	1.27 (inadequate)

Conclusions:

CBI was developed from an analysis of the behavioural and neuropsychiatric features which distinguish Alzheimer's disease (AD) from frontotemporal dementia (FTD) [3]. A revised version, CBI-R, has been published [25], and subscores of CBI to try to differentiate AD and FTD have also been examined [18].

LDM values for CBI were suboptimal (<1), as were SUI and NNSU, both parameters failing to achieve "adequate" classification.

The overall benefit of CBI may be in providing a structured behavioural symptom profile rather than a summated behavioural score.

References

1. Aji BM, Larner AJ. Cognitive assessment in an epilepsy clinic using AD8 questionnaire. Epilepsy Behav. 2018;85:234–6.
2. Amariglio RE, Donohue MC, Marshall GA, Rentz DM, Salmon DP, Ferris SH, et al. Tracking early decline in cognitive function in older individuals at risk for Alzheimer disease dementia: the Alzheimer's Disease Cooperative Study Cognitive Function Instrument. JAMA Neurol. 2015;72:446-54.
3. Bozeat S, Gregory CA, Lambon Ralph MA, Hodges JR. Which neuropsychiatric and behavioural features distinguish frontal and temporal variants of frontotemporal dementia from Alzheimer's disease? J Neurol Neurosurg Psychiatry. 2000;69:178–86.
4. Brodaty H, Pond D, Kemp NM, et al. The GPCOG: a new screening test for dementia designed for general practice. J Am Geriatr Soc. 2002;50:530–4.
5. Chen HH, Sun FJ, Yeh TL, Liu HE, Huang HL, Kuo BIT, Huang HY. The diagnostic accuracy of the Ascertain Dementia 8 questionnaire for detecting cognitive impairment in primary care in the community, clinics and hospitals: a systematic review and meta-analysis. Fam Pract. 2018;35:239–46.
6. Cherbuin N, Jorm AF. The IQCODE: using informant reports to assess cognitive change in the clinic and in older individuals living in the community. In: Larner AJ, editor. Cognitive screening instruments. A practical approach, 2nd ed. London: Springer;2017. p. 275–95.
7. Connon P, Larner A. Combining informant (AD8) and patient (MACE) cognitive screening. J Neurol Neurosurg Psychiatry. 2017;88(Suppl1):A20 (PO030).
8. Ehrensperger MM, Taylor KI, Berres M, Foldi NS, Dellenbach M, Bopp I, et al. BrainCheck – a very brief tool to detect incipient cognitive decline: optimized case-finding combining patient- and informant-based data. Alzheimers Res Ther. 2014;6:69.

9. Galvin JE, Goodyear M. Brief informant interviews to screen for dementia: the AD8 and Quick dementia rating system. In: Larner AJ, editor. Cognitive screening instruments. A practical approach, 2nd ed. London: Springer;2017. p. 297–312.

10. Galvin JE, Roe CM, Powlishta KK, et al. The AD8. A brief informant interview to detect dementia. Neurology. 2005;65:559–64.

11. Hancock P, Larner AJ. Cambridge Behavioural Inventory for the diagnosis of dementia. Prog Neurol Psychiatry. 2008;12(7):23–5.

12. Hancock P, Larner AJ. Diagnostic utility of the Informant Questionnaire on Cognitive Decline in the Elderly (IQCODE) and its combination with the Addenbrooke's Cognitive Examination-Revised (ACE-R) in a memory clinic-based population. Int Psychogeriatr. 2009;21:526-30.

13. Harrison JK, Fearon P, Noel-Storr AH, McShane R, Stott DJ, Quinn TJ. Informant Questionnaire on Cognitive Decline in the Elderly (IQCODE) for the diagnosis of dementia within a general practice (primary care) setting. Cochrane Database Syst Rev. 2014;CD010771.

14. Harrison JK, Fearon P, Noel-Storr AH, McShane R, Stott DJ, Quinn TJ. Informant Questionnaire on Cognitive Decline in the Elderly (IQCODE) for the diagnosis of dementia within a secondary care setting. Cochrane Database Syst Rev. 2015;CD010772.

15. Hendry K, Green C, McShane R, Noel-Storr AH, Stott DJ, Anwer S, Sutton AJ, Nurton JK, Quinn TJ. AD-8 for diagnosis of dementia across a variety of healthcare settings. Cochrane Database Syst Rev. 2019;3:CD011121.

16. Jorgensen K, Nielsen TR, Nielsen A, Waldorff FB, Hogh P, Jakobsen S, et al. Brief Assessment of Impaired Cognition (BASIC) – validation of a new dementia case-finding instrument integrating cognitive assessment with patient and informant report. Int J Geriatr Psychiatry. 2019;34:1724-33.

17. Jorm AF, Jacomb PA. The Informant Questionnaire on Cognitive Decline in the Elderly (IQCODE): socio-demographic correlates, reliability, validity and some norms. Psychol Med. 1989;19:1015-22.

18. Larner AJ. Cambridge Behavioural Inventory: diagnostic and differential diagnostic utility. J Neurol Neurosurg Psychiatry. 2008;79:351-2 (abstract 61).

19. Larner AJ. AD8 informant questionnaire for cognitive impairment: pragmatic diagnostic test accuracy study. J Geriatr Psychiatry Neurol. 2015;28:198–202.

20. Larner AJ. Dementia in clinical practice: a neurological perspective. Pragmatic studies in the Cognitive Function Clinic. 3rd edition. London: Springer; 2018, pp. 142-5.

21. National Institute for Health and Care Excellence. Dementia. Assessment, management and support for people living with dementia and their carers. NICE Guideline 97. Methods, evidence and recommendations. London: NICE;2018. https://www.nice.org.uk/guidance/ng97.

22. Quinn TJ, McShane R, Fearon P, Young C, Noel-Storr AH, Stott DJ. IQCODE for the diagnosis of Alzheimer's disease dementia and other dementias within a community setting. Cochrane Database Syst Rev. 2012;CD010079.

23. Seeher KM, Brodaty H. The General Practitioner Assessment of Cognition (GPCOG). In: Larner AJ (ed.). Cognitive screening instruments. A practical approach (2nd edition). London: Springer; 2017. p. 231-9.

24. Tsoi KK, Chan JY, Hirai HW, Wong SY, Kwok TC. Cognitive tests to detect dementia. A systematic review and meta-analysis. JAMA Intern Med. 2015;175:1450–8.

25. Wear HJ, Wedderburn CJ, Mioshi E, et al. The Cambridge Behavioural Inventory revised. Dement Neuropsychol. 2008;2:102-7.

26. Wedderburn C, Wear H, Brown J, et al. The utility of the Cambridge Behavioural Inventory in neurodegenerative disease. J Neurol Neurosurg Psychiatry. 2008;79:500–3.

27. Williamson JC, Larner AJ. Likelihood to be diagnosed or misdiagnosed: application to meta-analytic data for cognitive screening instruments. Neurodegener Dis Manag. 2019;9:91–5.

28. Ziso B, Larner AJ. AD8: Likelihood to diagnose or misdiagnose. J Neurol Neurosurg Psychiatry. 2019a;90:A20 (https://jnnp.bmj.com/content/90/12/A20.1).

Chapter 8
Depression Screeners

8.1 Introduction

Depression is an important differential diagnostic consideration in any patient presenting with cognitive complaints [10]. In addition, depression may be comorbid with dementia [12] and indeed may be a risk factor for the development of dementia [13]. Assessment of mood by means of brief depression screeners may therefore be indicated in the clinical encounter.

A number of instruments have been validated for identifying depression in dementia [6]. Patients scoring above threshold on these screeners may be candidates for treatment with anti-depressant medications.

8.2 Two-Question Depression Screener

Origin:
Arroll B, Khin N, Kerse N. Screening for depression in primary care with two verbally asked questions: cross sectional study. BMJ. 2003;327:1144–6 [3].

Content:
A two-question screener for depression, taking <1 min to perform. The patient is asked:
During the past month:

- Have you often been bothered by feeling down, depressed, or hopeless?
- Have you often been bothered by little interest or pleasure in doing things?

Data:
Categorical. If the patient answers yes to either one of these questions, he/she is coded as depressed.

© Springer Nature Switzerland AG 2020
A. J. Larner, *Manual of Screeners for Dementia*,
https://doi.org/10.1007/978-3-030-41636-2_8

Pragmatic studies:
Bharambe V, Larner AJ. Functional cognitive disorders: demographic and clinical features contribute to a positive diagnosis. Neurodegener Dis Manag. 2018;8:377–83 [4]. Elhadd K, Bharambe V, Larner AJ. Functional cognitive disorders: can sleep disturbance contribute to a positive diagnosis? J Sleep Disord Ther. 2018;7:291 [5].

Results
For diagnosis of functional cognitive disorders (FCD) versus cognitive disorder (dementia or MCI):

1. Demographics:

N	81
P = Prevalence of cognitive impairment (= pre-test probability)	0.44
Q = Level of the test = "Yes"	0.65

2. Paired measures of discrimination:

Sensitivity (Se), Specificity (Sp)	0.80, 0.53
PPV, NPV	0.68, 0.68
LR+, LR−	1.69 (slight), 0.38 (moderate)
CUI+, CUI−	0.54 (adequate), 0.358 (very poor)

3. Unitary measures of discrimination:

Accuracy	0.68
Y	0.33
PSI	0.36
SUI	0.90 (poor)

4. Numbers needed:

To diagnose (NND)	3.03
To predict (NNP)	2.78
To misdiagnose (NNM)	3.13
Likelihood to be diagnosed or misdiagnosed (LDM = NNM/NND, NNM/NNP)	1.03, 1.13
For screening utility (NNSU)	1.11 (inadequate)

Conclusions:
This two-question screener is very quick and easy to use. For the diagnosis of functional cognitive disorders the LDM>1 is encouraging but values for SUI and NNSU were inadequate.

Mood disturbance identified using this two-question screener for depression was more frequent in epilepsy patients with subjective memory complaint (SMC Likert Scale; Sect. 2.3) than those without [1].

8.3   Patient Health Questionnaire-9 (PHQ-9)

Origin:
Kroenke K, Spitzer RL, Williams JBW. The PHQ-9: validity of a brief depression severity measure. J Gen Intern Med. 2001;16:606–13 [11].

Content:
The Patient Health Questionnaire-9 (PHQ-9) is a brief validated instrument for measurement of the severity of depression, comprising a nine symptom checklist, with each symptom graded by frequency (score range 0–3) over the preceding two weeks.

• Little interest or pleasure in doing things
• Feeling down, depressed or hopeless
• Trouble falling or staying asleep or else sleeping too much
• Feeling tired or having little energy
• Poor appetite or overeating
• Feeling bad about self, a failure, have let self or family down
• Trouble concentrating (reading, TV)
• Moving or speaking so slowly that others have noticed; or fidgety, restless
• Thought you would be better off dead, or of hurting yourself

Data:
Quantitative, discrete, ordinal. Score range 0–27 (higher score = worse depression):

- 0–4: adjudged to indicate no depression
- 5–9: mild depression
- 10–14: moderate depression
- ≥15: severe depression.

May be used categorically, e.g. any score ≥10 indicating consideration of the need for trial of antidepressant medication.

Pragmatic studies:
Hancock P, Larner AJ. Clinical utility of Patient Health Questionnaire-9 (PHQ-9) in memory clinics. Int J Psychiatry Clin Pract. 2009;13:188–91 [7].

Results
For diagnosis of dementia, cut-off ≤9/27 (defined by optimal accuracy):

1. Demographics:

N	113
P = Prevalence of cognitive impairment (= pre-test probability)	0.43
Q = Level of the test	0.69

2. Paired measures of discrimination:

Sensitivity (Se), Specificity (Sp)	0.86, 0.44
PPV, NPV	0.54, 0.80
LR+, LR−	1.52 (slight), 0.32 (moderate)
CUI+, CUI−	0.46 (poor), 0.35 (very poor)

3. Unitary measures of discrimination:

Accuracy	0.62
Y	0.30
PSI	0.34
SUI	0.81 (poor)

4. Numbers needed:

To diagnose (NND)	3.33
To predict (NNP)	2.94
To misdiagnose (NNM)	2.63
Likelihood to be diagnosed or misdiagnosed (LDM = NNM/NND, NNM/NNP)	0.79, 0.89
For screening utility (NNSU)	1.23 (inadequate)

Conclusions:
Although the mean PHQ-9 scores differed between the demented and non-demented groups (4.1 ± 5.4 versus 7.1 ± 7.9, $p<0.01$), nevertheless PHQ-9 showed poor metrics for dementia diagnosis (LDM < 1, SUI and NNSU

inadequate), perhaps unsurprisingly for an instrument designed to screen for depression. However, a score>9/27 in patients attending a memory clinic might be taken as an indicator of the need to consider depression and possibly treatment with an antidepressant.

A meta-analysis found a PHQ-9 cut-off score of 10 or above maximised sensitivity and specificity for the diagnosis of major depression [9].

8.4 Cornell Scale for Depression in Dementia (CSDD)

Origin:
Alexopoulos GS, Abrams RC, Young RC, Shamoian CA. Cornell Scale for Depression in Dementia. Biol Psych. 1988;23:271–84 [2].

Content:
The Cornell Scale for Depression in Dementia (CSDD) is a 19-item instrument based on both patient and informant interview, with each item rated for severity, ranging from 0 to 2 (absent to severe).

Data:
Quantitative, discrete, ordinal. Score range 0–38 (higher score = worse depression):

- <6: absence of significant depressive symptoms
- >10: probable major depressive episode
- >18: definite major depressive episode.

May be used categorically, e.g. any score ≥6 or >10 indicating consideration of the need for trial of antidepressant medication.

Pragmatic studies:
Hancock P, Larner AJ. Cornell Scale for Depression in Dementia: clinical utility in a memory clinic. Int J Psychiatry Clin Pract. 2015;19:71−4 [8].

Results
For diagnosis of dementia, cut-off ≤5/38 (defined by optimal accuracy):

1. Demographics:

N	242
P = Prevalence of cognitive impairment (= pre-test probability)	0.405
Q = Level of the test	0.66

2. Paired measures of discrimination:

Sensitivity (Se), Specificity (Sp)	0.80, 0.43
PPV, NPV	0.49, 0.76
LR+, LR−	1.40 (slight), 0.47 (moderate)
CUI+, CUI−	0.39 (poor), 0.33 (very poor)

3. Unitary measures of discrimination:

Accuracy	0.59
Y	0.23
PSI	0.24
SUI	0.72 (poor)

4. Numbers needed:

To diagnose (NND)	4.35
To predict (NNP)	4.17
To misdiagnose (NNM)	2.44
Likelihood to be diagnosed or misdiagnosed (LDM = NNM/NND, NNM/NNP)	0.56, 0.69
For screening utility (NNSU)	1.39 (inadequate)

Conclusions:

Although the mean CSDD scores differed between the demented and non-demented groups (3.2 ± 4.2 versus 5.3 ± 5.9, $p < 0.01$), nevertheless CSDD showed poor metrics for dementia diagnosis (LDM<1, SUI and NNSU inadequate), perhaps unsurprisingly for a depression screener. However, a score >5/38 in patients attending a memory clinic might be taken as an indicator of the need to consider depression and possibly treatment with an antidepressant.

Goodarzi et al. [6] identified CSDD as one of the two most sensitive scales for identifying depression in patients with dementia in an outpatient setting.

References

1. Aji BM, Elhadd K, Larner AJ. Cognitive symptoms in people with epilepsy: role of sleep and mood disturbance. J Sleep Disord Ther. 2019;8:1.
2. Alexopoulos GS, Abrams RC, Young RC, Shamoian CA. Cornell Scale for Depression in Dementia. Biol Psych. 1988;23:271–84.

3. Arroll B, Khin N, Kerse N. Screening for depression in primary care with two verbally asked questions: cross sectional study. BMJ. 2003;327:1144–6.
4. Bharambe V, Larner AJ. Functional cognitive disorders: demographic and clinical features contribute to a positive diagnosis. Neurodegener Dis Manag. 2018;8:377–83.
5. Elhadd K, Bharambe V, Larner AJ. Functional cognitive disorders: can sleep disturbance contribute to a positive diagnosis? J Sleep Disord Ther. 2018;7:291.
6. Goodarzi ZS, Mele BS, Roberts DJ, Holroyd-Leduc J. Depression case finding in individuals with dementia: a systematic review and meta-analysis. J Am Geriatr Soc. 2017;65:937–48.
7. Hancock P, Larner AJ. Clinical utility of Patient Health Questionnaire-9 (PHQ-9) in memory clinics. Int J Psychiatry Clin Pract. 2009;13:188-91.
8. Hancock P, Larner AJ. Cornell Scale for Depression in Dementia: clinical utility in a memory clinic. Int J Psychiatry Clin Pract. 2015;19:71-4.
9. Levis B, Benedetti A, Thombs BD; DEPRESsion Screening Data (DEPRESSD) Collaboration. Accuracy of Patient Health Questionnaire-9 (PHQ-9) for screening to detect major depression: individual participant data meta-analysis. BMJ. 2019;365:l1476.
10. Knapskog AB, Barca ML, Engedal K. Prevalence of depression among memory clinic patients as measured by the Cornell Scale of Depression in Dementia. Aging Mental Health. 2014;18:579-87.
11. Kroenke K, Spitzer RL, Williams JBW. The PHQ-9: validity of a brief depression severity measure. J Gen Intern Med. 2001;16:606–13.
12. Lundquist RS, Bernens A, Olsen CG. Comorbid disease in geriatric patients: dementia and depression. Am Fam Physician. 1997;55:2687-94, 2703-4.
13. Mirza SS, Wolters FJ, Swanson SA, et al. 10-year trajectories of depressive symptoms and risk of dementia: a population-based study. Lancet Psychiatry. 2016;3:628–35.

Chapter 9
Functional Screeners

9.1 Introduction

It may be patient function rather than cognition per se that impacts most on patients and, especially, carers and hence on decisions regarding nursing home placement. Thus some assessment of overall function, based on activities of daily living, may be indicated, as well as cognitive assessment, in patients with cognitive complaints. A number of scales are available for this purpose [9, 10] although both their utility and exact place in dementia assessment remain to be precisely defined.

The possibility that a combination of functional and cognitive scales might improve screening utility is attractive since dementia typically impairs both domains, although factors other than dementia severity may influence functional capacity. Scales assessing both cognition and function have been described [5], including Free-Cog (Sect. 6.7). Combining functional and cognitive scales is addressed in Chap. 12 [7].

9.2 Instrumental Activities of Daily Living (IADL) Scale

Origin:
Lawton MP, Brody EM. Assessment of older people: self-maintaining and instrumental activities of daily living. Gerontologist. 1969;9:179–86 [8].

Content:
The Instrumental Activities of Daily Living (IADL) Scale assesses six basic ADLs (also known as the Physical Self-Maintenance Scale) and eight instrumental ADLs in a hierarchical manner according to degree of autonomy. Patients may require the assistance of an informant to complete the scale.

© Springer Nature Switzerland AG 2020
A. J. Larner, *Manual of Screeners for Dementia*,
https://doi.org/10.1007/978-3-030-41636-2_9

Instrumental ADL:
Ability to use telephone Shopping Food preparation Housekeeping Laundry Mode of transportation Responsibility for own medications Ability to handle finances
Basic ADL (= Physical Self-Maintenance Scale)
Toileting Feeding Dressing Grooming Physical ambulation Bathing

A derivative, shortened form, the 4-IADL, has also been described [1].

Data:
Quantitative, discrete, ordinal. Scoring of each ADL domain is by forced choice, either 0 (dependent) or 1 (independent), giving a score range of 0–14 (impaired to normal).

Pragmatic studies:
Hancock P, Larner AJ. The diagnosis of dementia: diagnostic accuracy of an instrument measuring activities of daily living in a clinic-based population. Dement Geriatr Cogn Disord. 2007;23:133–9 [3].

Results
For diagnosis of dementia, cut-off ≤13/14 (defined by optimal accuracy):

1. Demographics:

N	296
P = Prevalence of dementia (= pre-test probability)	0.52
Q = Level of the test	0.69

2. Paired measures of discrimination:

Sensitivity (Se), Specificity (Sp)	0.87, 0.50
PPV, NPV	0.65, 0.78
LR+, LR−	1.74 (slight), 0.26 (moderate)
CUI+, CUI−	0.57 (adequate), 0.39 (poor)

3. Unitary measures of discrimination:

Accuracy	0.69
Y	0.37
PSI	0.43
SUI	0.96 (poor)

4. Numbers needed:

To diagnose (NND)	2.70
To predict (NNP)	2.33
To misdiagnose (NNM)	3.23
Likelihood to be diagnosed or misdiagnosed (NNM/NND, NNM/NNP)	1.19, 1.39
For screening utility (NNSU)	1.04 (inadequate)

Conclusions:

The IADL Scale has only modest diagnostic utility for dementia, in part because of a ceiling effect, with many cognitively impaired patients scoring highly (i.e. normal).

Although LDM >1 is encouraging, the values for SUI and NNSU were inadequate.

Use of functional scales to assist in differential diagnosis of dementia, specifically of Alzheimer's disease from frontotemporal dementia (with the latter more functionally impaired in ADL), has been reported. However, analysis of these patient subgroups from this study [6] did not show statistically significant differences in IADL or 4-IADL [1] scores.

The combination of IADL Scale with cognitive screening instruments (MMSE, ACE-R) has also been examined (Sects. 12.4 and 12.5 respectively).

9.3   Zarit Burden Interview (ZBI)

Origin:

Zarit SH, Reever KE, Bach-Peterson J. Relatives of the impaired elderly: correlates of feelings of burden. Gerontologist. 1980;20:649–55 [12].

Content:

Originally described as a 29-item instrument. A number of other ZBI versions have subsequently been published, including full (22 items), short (12 items), and screening (4 items) versions [2, 4, 13].

Data:
Quantitative, discrete, ordinal. Statements are ranked by the informant as occurring Never, Rarely, Sometimes, Quite frequently, or Nearly always, with these responses scoring 0–4 respectively. For the full (22 item) ZBI, score range = 0–88 (low burden to high burden), classified as:

- 0–21: little or no burden.
- 21–40: mild to moderate burden.
- 41–60: moderate to severe burden.
- 61–88: severe burden.

Hence scores might be dichotomised as >40 regarded as high burden, ≤40 low burden.

Pragmatic studies:
Stagg B, Larner AJ. Zarit Burden Interview: pragmatic study in a dedicated cognitive function clinic. Prog Neurol Psychiatry. 2015;19(4):23–7 [11].

Results
For any cognitive impairment, cut-off >40/88:

1. Demographics:

N	45
P = Prevalence of cognitive impairment (= pre-test probability)	0.69
Q = Level of the test	0.29

2. Paired measures of discrimination:

Sensitivity (Se), Specificity (Sp)	0.32, 0.79
PPV, NPV	0.77, 0.34
LR+, LR−	1.51 (slight), 0.86 (slight)
CUI+, CUI−	0.25 (very poor), 0.27 (very poor)

3. Unitary measures of discrimination:

Accuracy	0.47
Y	0.11
PSI	0.11
SUI	0.52 (very poor)

4. Numbers needed:

To diagnose (NND)	9.23
To predict (NNP)	8.85
To misdiagnose (NNM)	1.88
Likelihood to be diagnosed or misdiagnosed (NNM/ NND, NNM/NNP)	0.20, 0.21
For screening utility (NNSU)	1.92 (inadequate)

Conclusions:
Although a small study, the data provide no evidence to suggest a diagnostic role for ZBI. LDM, SUI and NNSU were all inadequate. Just as inferences about caregiver burden cannot be based on patient cognitive scores, scores on caregiver burden cannot be used as a surrogate for cognitive status.

References

1. Barberger-Gateau P, Commenges D, Gagnon M, Letenneur L, Sauvel C, Dartigues JF. Instrumental activities of daily living as a screening tool for cognitive impairment and dementia in elderly community dwellers. J Am Geriatr Soc. 1992;40:1129–34.
2. Bédard M, Molloy DW, Squire L, Dubois S, Lever JA, O'Donnell M. The Zarit Burden Interview: a new short version and screening version. Gerontologist. 2001;41:652–7.
3. Hancock P, Larner AJ. The diagnosis of dementia: diagnostic accuracy of an instrument measuring activities of daily living in a clinic-based population. Dement Geriatr Cogn Disord. 2007;23:133–9.
4. Hebert R, Bravo G, Preville M. Reliability, validity and reference values of the Zarit Burden Interview for assessing informal caregivers of community-dwelling older persons with dementia. Can J Aging. 2000;19:494–507.
5. Heller S, Mendoza Rebolledo C, Rodriguez Blazquez C, Carrasco Chillon L, Perez Munoz A, Rodriguez Perez A, et al. Validation of the multimodal assessment of capacities in severe dementia: a novel cognitive and functional scale for use in severe dementia. J Neurol. 2015;262:1198–208.
6. Larner AJ, Hancock P. Activities of daily living in frontotemporal dementia and Alzheimer disease. Neurology. 2008;70:658.
7. Larner AJ, Hancock P. Does combining cognitive and functional scales facilitate the diagnosis of dementia? Int J Geriatr Psychiatry. 2012;27:547–8.
8. Lawton MP, Brody EM. Assessment of older people: self-maintaining and instrumental activities of daily living. Gerontologist. 1969;9:179–86.
9. Marshall GA, Amariglio RE, Sperling RA, Rentz DM. Activities of daily living: where do they fit in the diagnosis of Alzheimer's disease? Neurodegener Dis Manag. 2012;2:483–91.
10. Sikkes SAM, de Lange-de Klerk ESM, Pijnenburg YAL, Scheltens P, Uitdehaag BMJ. A systematic review of Instrumental Activities of Daily Living Scales in dementia: room for improvement. J Neurol Neurosurg Psychiatry. 2009;80:7–12.

11. Stagg B, Larner AJ. Zarit Burden Interview: pragmatic study in a dedicated cognitive function clinic. Prog Neurol Psychiatry. 2015;19(4):23–7.
12. Zarit SH, Reever KE, Bach-Peterson J. Relatives of the impaired elderly: correlates of feelings of burden. Gerontologist. 1980;20:649-55.
13. Zarit SH, Orr NK, Zarit JM. The hidden victims of Alzheimer's disease: Families under stress. New York: New York University Press; 1985.

Chapter 10
Sleep Disorder Screeners

10.1   Introduction

The interactions between sleep, cognitive function, and dementia are subjects of much ongoing research. The relationship between Alzheimer's disease (AD) and sleep disturbance may be bidirectional: disturbed sleep may be a consequence of AD (a particularly challenging symptom for caregivers) and sleep disturbance may increase the risk of AD through increased production of amyloid peptides and neuroinflammatory processes [9]. The amount of sleep required for optimal cognitive performance remains constant regardless of age, but older people sleep less, suggesting that more sleep may be a good idea as we age [14].

Sleep disturbance is common in patients attending cognitive disorders and memory clinics and so should be looked for, an inquiry which may be facilitated with the use of sleep screeners. In addition to the instruments examined in pragmatic studies and described here, other sleep screeners are available. The Neuropsychiatric Inventory (NPI; [6]) has an item devoted to sleep which was subsequently expanded into the Sleep Disorders Inventory (SDI; [16]) which may be used to assess and quantify sleep disturbance in dementia patients [5].

Other sleep screeners looking for specific sleep disorders may also be subjected to pragmatic studies, such as the STOP-Bang [4] for obstructive sleep apnoea [12, 17], and the REM Sleep Behaviour Screening Questionnaire (RBDSQ; [15]) for REM Sleep Behaviour Disorder in suspected or established synucleinopathies [18].

10.2   Jenkins Sleep Questionnaire (JSQ)

Origin:
Jenkins CD, Stanton BA, Niemcryk SJ, Rose RM. A scale for the estimation of sleep problems in clinical research. J Clin Epidemiol. 1988;41:313–21 [10].

Content:
This scale addresses four sleep-related symptoms over the previous four week period. The patient is asked:
During the previous 4 weeks have you experienced:

- Difficulty falling asleep?
- Waking up several times per night?
- Difficulty staying asleep (including waking up too early)?
- Waking up feeling tired and worn out after usual amount of sleep?

If yes is answered to any one of these, a frequency question is then asked: occurring 15 or more nights over the four week period? A dichotomous index (JSQ+, JSQ−) is easily computed if the respondent reports that any of the sleep disturbances occurred on 15 or more nights during the previous 4 weeks [11].

Data:
Categorical when dichotomised.

Pragmatic studies:
Bharambe V, Larner AJ. Functional cognitive disorders: demographic and clinical features contribute to a positive diagnosis. Neurodegener Dis Manag. 2018;8:377–83 [2].
Elhadd K, Bharambe V, Larner AJ. Functional cognitive disorders: can sleep disturbance contribute to a positive diagnosis? J Sleep Disord Ther. 2018;7:291 [7].

Results
For diagnosis of functional cognitive disorders (FCD) versus cognitive disorder (dementia or MCI):

1. Demographics:

N	84
P = Prevalence of cognitive impairment (= pre-test probability)	0.43
Q = Level of the test	0.69

2. Paired measures of discrimination:

Sensitivity (Se), Specificity (Sp)	0.83, 0.50
PPV, NPV	0.69, 0.69

| LR+, LR− | 1.67 (slight), 0.33 (moderate) |
| CUI+, CUI− | 0.57 (adequate), 0.35 (very poor) |

3. Unitary measures of discrimination:

Accuracy	0.69
Y	0.33
PSI	0.38
SUI	0.92 (poor)

4. Numbers needed:

To diagnose (NND)	3.00
To predict (NNP)	2.62
To misdiagnose (NNM)	3.23
Likelihood to be diagnosed or misdiagnosed (LDM = NNM/NND, NNM/NNP)	1.08, 1.23
For screening utility (NNSU)	1.09 (inadequate)

Conclusions:

The Jenkins Sleep Questionnaire or Scale is very quick (administration time ca. 1 minute) and easy to use and score. Its brevity (four items) cannot address the spectrum of sleep disorders and hence it can only be used as a preliminary screener [13]. Dichotomising the test results in loss of statistical power [11], although generally clinicians prefer tests which can be easily categorised in practice.

For the diagnosis of functional cognitive disorders the LDM > 1 is encouraging but values for SUI and NNSU were inadequate.

Sleep disturbance identified using JSQ was more frequent in epilepsy patients with subjective memory complaint (SMC Likert Scale; Sect. 2.3) than those without [1].

10.3   Pittsburgh Sleep Quality Index (PSQI)

Origin:

Buysse DJ, Reynolds CF 3rd, Monk TH, Berman SR, Kupfer DJ. The Pittsburgh Sleep Quality Index: a new instrument for psychiatric practice and research. Psychiatry Res. 1989;28:193–213 [3].

Content:

A self-rated questionnaire which assesses sleep quality and disturbances over a 1-month period to generate seven component scores (range 0–3) and one global score (range 0–21).

Data:

Quantitative, discrete, ordinal. Score range 0–21, normal to impaired (i.e. lower scores better sleep quality).

Pragmatic studies:

Hancock P, Larner AJ. Diagnostic utility of the Pittsburgh sleep quality index in memory clinics. Int J Geriatr Psychiatry. 2009;24:1237–41 [8].

Results

For diagnosis of dementia versus no dementia, cut-off ≤5/21 (from index study):

1. Demographics:

N	310
P = Prevalence of cognitive impairment (= pre-test probability)	0.50
Q = Level of the test	0.53

2. Paired measures of discrimination:

Sensitivity (Se), Specificity (Sp)	0.66, 0.60
PPV, NPV	0.62, 0.64
LR+, LR−	1.66 (slight), 0.56 (slight)
CUI+, CUI−	0.41 (poor), 0.38 (poor)

3. Unitary measures of discrimination:

Accuracy	0.63
Y	0.26
PSI	0.26
SUI	0.79 (poor)

4. Numbers needed:

To diagnose (NND)	3.85
To predict (NNP)	3.85
To misdiagnose (NNM)	2.70

Likelihood to be diagnosed or misdiagnosed (LDM = NNM/NND, NNM/NNP)	0.70, 0.70
For screening utility (NNSU)	1.27 (inadequate)

Conclusions:

Although PSQI is a longer instrument than JSQ in terms of administration and scoring time, it may be argued that, like JSQ, it does not address the spectrum of sleep disorders and hence can only be used as a preliminary screener.

The unitary metrics indicate inadequacy for dementia diagnosis. However, PSQI may have pragmatic use in identifying cognitive clinic attenders with poor sleep quality, the risk of which was found to be higher in non-demented individuals. Some of these individuals may have functional cognitive disorders [7] and may benefit cognitively from interventions to improve their sleep.

References

1. Aji BM, Elhadd K, Larner AJ. Cognitive symptoms in people with epilepsy: role of sleep and mood disturbance. J Sleep Disord Ther. 2019;8:1.
2. Bharambe V, Larner AJ. Functional cognitive disorders: demographic and clinical features contribute to a positive diagnosis. Neurodegener Dis Manag. 2018;8:377–83.
3. Buysse DJ, Reynolds CF 3rd, Monk TH, Berman SR, Kupfer DJ. The Pittsburgh Sleep Quality Index: a new instrument for psychiatric practice and research. Psychiatry Res. 1989;28:193–213.
4. Chung F, Subramanyam R, Liao P, et al. High STOP-Bang score indicates a high probability of obstructive sleep apnoea. Br J Anaesth. 2012;108:768–75.
5. Culshaw M, Larner AJ. Assessing the impact of sleep disorders on people with dementia and their caregivers. J Dement Care. 2009;17(5):38.
6. Cummings JL, Mega MS, Gray K, et al. The Neuropsychiatric Inventory: comprehensive assessment of psychopathology in dementia. Neurology. 1994;44:2308–14.
7. Elhadd K, Bharambe V, Larner AJ. Functional cognitive disorders: can sleep disturbance contribute to a positive diagnosis? J Sleep Disord Ther. 2018;7:291.
8. Hancock P, Larner AJ. Diagnostic utility of the Pittsburgh Sleep Quality Index in memory clinics. Int J Geriatr Psychiatry. 2009;24:1237–41.
9. Irwin MR, Vitiello MV. Implications of sleep disturbance and inflammation for Alzheimer's disease dementia. Lancet Neurol. 2019;18:296–306.
10. Jenkins CD, Stanton BA, Niemcryk SJ, Rose RM. A scale for the estimation of sleep problems in clinical research. J Clin Epidemiol. 1988;41:313–21.
11. Lallukka T, Dregan A, Armstrong D. Comparison of a sleep item from the General Health Questionnaire-12 with the Jenkins Sleep Questionnaire as measures of sleep disturbance. J Epidemiol. 2011; 21:474–80.
12. Larner AJ, Ziso B. Screening for obstructive sleep apnoea using the STOPBANG questionnaire. Clin Med. 2018;18:108–9.
13. Shahid A, Wilkinson K, Marcu S, Shapiro CM. Jenkins Sleep Scale. In: Shahid A, Wilkinson K, Marcu S, Shapiro CM (eds). STOP, THAT and one hundred other sleep scales. New York: Springer, 2011:203–4.
14. Sternin A, Burns A, Owen AM. Thirty-five years of computerized cognitive assessment of aging – where are we now? Diagnostics (Basel). 2019;9:E114.

15. Stiasny-Kolster K, Mayer G, Schafer S, Moller JC, Heinzel-Gutenbrunner M, Oertel WH. The REM Sleep Behavior Disorder Screening Questionnaire – a new diagnostic instrument. Mov Disord. 2007;22:2386–93.
16. Tractenberg RE, Singer CM, Cummings JL, Thal LJ. The Sleep Disorders Inventory: an instrument for studies of sleep disturbance in persons with Alzheimer's disease. J Sleep Res. 2003;12:331–7.
17. Ziso B, Larner AJ. STOP-Bang: screening for obstructive sleep apnoea in a cognitive disorders clinic. J Sleep Disord Ther. 2016a;5:223.
18. Ziso B, Larner A. REM sleep behaviour screening questionnaire (RBDSQ): validation study. Eur J Neurol. 2016b;23(Suppl1):240 (abstract P11273).

Chapter 11
Combining Screeners (1): Cognitive Screeners

11.1 Introduction

Tests may be combined using simple logical rules, either in series or in parallel. In series combination (also known as the "And" rule, conjunctive combination, or "believe the negative") both tests are required to be positive for the target diagnosis to be made. In parallel combination (also known as the "Or" rule, compensatory combination, or "believe the positive") either test positive is sufficient for the target diagnosis to be made [9, 14, 15].

Generally it is found that, for paired measures, series combination improves specificity, PPV, and LR+ at the expense of sensitivity, NPV, and LR−, all of which are generally better in the parallel combination.

The effect of series and parallel combination on LDM, SUI, and various number needed metrics has not, to my knowledge, been examined hitherto. In this chapter combinations of cognitive screeners are examined; other combinations form the subject of Chap. 12.

Recommendations for the detection of dementia from both the Alzheimer Association [3] and the International Association of Gerontology and Geriatrics [17] suggest combined use of a patient performance measurement and an informant interview. Patient-based cognitive scales and informant-based questionnaires may test different constructs, an asymmetry which might afford additional diagnostic information.

© Springer Nature Switzerland AG 2020
A. J. Larner, *Manual of Screeners for Dementia*,
https://doi.org/10.1007/978-3-030-41636-2_11

11.2   MMSE and MoCA

Origins:
MMSE:
Folstein MF, Folstein SE, McHugh PR. Mini-Mental State. A practical method for grading the cognitive state of patients for the clinician. J Psychiatr Res. 1975;12:189–98 [4].
NB: Copyright Psychological Assessment Resources
MoCA:
Nasreddine ZS, Phillips NA, Bédirian V, Charbonneau S, Whitehead V, Collin I, et al. The Montreal Cognitive Assessment, MoCA: a brief screening tool for mild cognitive impairment. J Am Geriatr Soc. 2005;53:695–9 [18].

Contents:
Details on the item content of MMSE and MoCA may be found in Sects. 5.2 and 6.5 respectively.

Data:
Both: Quantitative, discrete, ordinal. Score range 0–30, impaired to normal.

Pragmatic studies:
Larner AJ. Screening utility of the Montreal Cognitive Assessment (MoCA): in place of—or as well as—the MMSE? Int Psychogeriatr. 2012;24:391–6 [10].

Results
For diagnosis of any cognitive impairment:

1. Demographics:

N	150
P = Prevalence of cognitive impairment (= pre-test probability)	0.43
Q = Levels of the tests for cognitive impairment	MMSE 0.37, MoCA 0.67

2. Paired measures of discrimination:

	Series: MoCA ≥26/30 and MMSE ≥26/30	Parallel: MoCA ≥26/30 or MMSE ≥26/30
Sensitivity (Se), Specificity (Sp)	0.65, 0.92	0.97, 0.59
PPV, NPV	0.85, 0.78	0.64, 0.96
LR+, LR−	7.90 (large), 0.38 (moderate)	2.35 (moderate), 0.05 (very large)
CUI+, CUI−	0.56 (adequate), 0.72 (good)	0.62 (adequate), 0.57 (adequate)

3. Unitary measures of discrimination:

	Series: MoCA ≥26/30 and MMSE ≥26/30	Parallel: MoCA ≥26/30 or MMSE ≥26/30
Accuracy	0.80	0.75
Y	0.57	0.56
PSI	0.63	0.60
SUI	1.28 (good)	1.19 (adequate)

4. Numbers needed:

	Series: MoCA ≥26/30 and MMSE ≥26/30	Parallel: MoCA ≥26/30 or MMSE ≥26/30
To diagnose (NND)	1.75	1.79
To predict (NNP)	1.59	1.67
To misdiagnose (NNM)	5.00	4.00
Likelihood to be diagnosed or misdiagnosed (NNM/NND, NNM/NNP)	2.86, 3.15	2.23, 2.40
For screening utility (NNSU)	0.78 (good)	0.84 (adequate)

Conclusions:

As anticipated, series combination of MMSE and MoCA improved specificity, PPV, and LR+ at the expense of sensitivity, NPV, and LR−, all of which were better in the parallel combination.

LDM, SUI, and NNSU were all good for the series combination (SUI and NNSU were on the threshold of excellent), but only adequate in the parallel combination. These data suggest a better balance in the series combination, but if avoidance of false negatives is key for clinicians then the high sensitivity of the parallel combination may be preferred, despite inferior LDM, SUI, and NNSU.

11.3   MMSE and IQCODE

Origins:

MMSE:

Folstein MF, Folstein SE, McHugh PR. Mini-Mental State. A practical method for grading the cognitive state of patients for the clinician. J Psychiatr Res. 1975;12:189–98 [4].

NB: Copyright Psychological Assessment Resources
IQCODE:
Jorm AF, Jacomb PA. The Informant Questionnaire on Cognitive Decline in the Elderly (IQCODE): socio-demographic correlates, reliability, validity and some norms. Psychol Med. 1989;19:1015–22 [8].

Contents:
Details on the item content of MMSE and IQCODE may be found in Sects. 5.2 and 7.3 respectively.

Data:
MMSE: Quantitative, discrete, ordinal. Score range 0–30, impaired to normal.

IQCODE: Quantitative, discrete, ordinal. Score range = 1–5, higher scores suggest greater impairment.

Pragmatic studies:
Hancock P, Larner AJ. Diagnostic utility of the Informant Questionnaire on Cognitive Decline in the Elderly (IQCODE) and its combination with the Addenbrooke's Cognitive Examination-Revised (ACE-R) in a memory clinic-based population. Int Psychogeriatr. 2009;21:526–30 [6].

Results
For diagnosis of dementia:

1. Demographics:

N	132
P = Prevalence of dementia (= pre-test probability)	0.55
Q = Levels of the tests for cognitive impairment	MMSE 0.45, IQCODE 0.77

2. Paired measures of discrimination:

	Series: IQCODE ≥3.6/5 and MMSE <24/30	Parallel: IQCODE ≥3.6/5 or MMSE <24/30
Sensitivity (Se), Specificity (Sp)	0.64, 0.88	0.95, 0.36
PPV, NPV	0.87, 0.67	0.64, 0.84
LR+, LR−	5.43 (large), 0.40 (moderate)	1.47 (slight), 0.15 (large)
CUI+, CUI−	0.56 (adequate), 0.59 (adequate)	0.61 (adequate), 0.30 (very poor)

3. Unitary measures of discrimination:

	Series: IQCODE ≥3.6/5 and MMSE <24/30	Parallel: IQCODE ≥3.6/5 or MMSE <24/30
Accuracy	0.75	0.68
Y	0.52	0.31
PSI	0.54	0.48
SUI	1.15 (adequate)	0.91 (poor)

4. Numbers needed:

	Series: IQCODE ≥3.6/5 and MMSE <24/30	Parallel: IQCODE ≥3.6/5 or MMSE <24/30
To diagnose (NND)	1.92	3.23
To predict (NNP)	1.85	2.08
To misdiagnose (NNM)	4.00	3.13
Likelihood to be diagnosed or misdiagnosed (NNM/NND, NNM/NNP)	2.08, 2.16	0.97, 1.50
For screening utility (NNSU)	0.87 (adequate)	1.10 (inadequate)

Conclusions:

The pattern of results combining patient-performance (MMSE) and informant (IQCODE) scales was similar to that seen combining two patient-performance scales (MMSE and MoCA; Sect. 11.2), namely better specificity, PPV, and LR+ at the expense of sensitivity, NPV, and LR− in the series as compared to the parallel combination.

LDM, SUI, and NNSU were all adequate for the series combination but inferior in the parallel combination. The high sensitivity and NPV of the latter combination appears to be its only recommendation.

11.4   MMSE and AD8

Origins:
MMSE:
Folstein MF, Folstein SE, McHugh PR. Mini-Mental State. A practical method for grading the cognitive state of patients for the clinician. J Psychiatr Res. 1975;12:189–98 [4].
NB: Copyright Psychological Assessment Resources
AD8:
Galvin JE, Roe CM, Powlishta KK, et al. The AD8. A brief informant interview to detect dementia. Neurology. 2005;65:559–64 [5].

Contents:
Details on the item content of MMSE and AD8 may be found in Sects. 5.2 and 7.2 respectively.

Data:
MMSE: Quantitative, discrete, ordinal. Score range 0–30, impaired to normal.
AD8: Quantitative, discrete, ordinal. Score range 8–0, impaired to normal (i.e. negatively scored).

Pragmatic studies:
Larner AJ. AD8 informant questionnaire for cognitive impairment: pragmatic diagnostic test accuracy study. J Geriatr Psychiatry Neurol. 2015;28:198–202 [11].

Results
For diagnosis of any cognitive impairment:

1. Demographics:

N	125
P = Prevalence of cognitive impairment (= pre-test probability)	0.56
Q = Levels of the tests for cognitive impairment	MMSE 0.41, AD8 0.92

2. Paired measures of discrimination:

	Series: AD8 ≥2/8 and MMSE ≤24/30	Parallel: AD8 ≥2/8 or MMSE ≤24/30
Sensitivity (Se), Specificity (Sp)	0.50, 0.83	1.00, 0.08
PPV, NPV	0.80, 0.55	0.60, 1.00
LR+, LR−	2.94 (moderate), 0.60 (slight)	1.08 (slight), 0 (very large)
CUI+, CUI−	0.40 (poor), 0.46 (poor)	0.60 (adequate), 0.08 (very poor)

3. Unitary measures of discrimination:

	Series: AD8≥2/8 and MMSE ≤24/30	Parallel: AD8 ≥2/8 or MMSE ≤24/30
Accuracy	0.64	0.61
Y	0.33	0.08
PSI	0.35	0.60
SUI	0.86 (poor)	0.68 (very poor)

4. Numbers needed:

	Series: AD8 ≥2/8 and MMSE ≤24/30	Parallel: AD8 ≥2/8 or MMSE ≤24/30
To diagnose (NND)	3.03	12.5
To predict (NNP)	2.86	1.67
To misdiagnose (NNM)	2.78	2.56
Likelihood to be diag- nosed or misdiagnosed (NNM/NND, NNM/NNP)	0.92, 0.97	0.21, 1.54
For screening utility (NNSU)	1.16 (inadequate)	1.47 (inadequate)

Conclusions:

This combination of patient-performance (MMSE) and informant (AD8) scales showed less impressive results than a similar combination (MMSE and IQCODE; Sect. 11.3), although the pattern of better specificity, PPV, and LR+ in the series as compared to the parallel combination was maintained.

LDM, SUI, and NNSU were all suboptimal or inadequate for both the series and parallel combinations. This is probably related to the very poor specificity of the AD8 in isolation (Sect. 7.2).

11.5   ACE-R and IQCODE

Origins:

ACE-R:

Mioshi E, Dawson K, Mitchell J, Arnold R, Hodges JR. The Addenbrooke's Cognitive Examination Revised: a brief cognitive test battery for dementia screening. Int J Geriatr Psychiatry. 2006;21:1078–85 [16].

IQCODE:

Jorm AF, Jacomb PA. The Informant Questionnaire on Cognitive Decline in the Elderly (IQCODE): socio-demographic correlates, reliability, validity and some norms. Psychol Med. 1989;19:1015–22 [8].

Contents:

Details on the item content of ACE-R and IQCODE may be found in Sects. 6.3 and 7.3 respectively.

Data:

ACE-R: Quantitative, discrete, ordinal. Score range 0–100, impaired to normal.

IQCODE: Quantitative, discrete, ordinal. Score range = 1–5, higher scores suggest greater impairment.

Pragmatic studies:

Hancock P, Larner AJ. Diagnostic utility of the Informant Questionnaire on Cognitive Decline in the Elderly (IQCODE) and its combination with the Addenbrooke's Cognitive Examination-Revised (ACE-R) in a memory clinic-based population. Int Psychogeriatr. 2009;21:526–30 [6].

Results
For diagnosis of dementia:

1. Demographics:

N	114
P = Prevalence of dementia (= pre-test probability)	0.51
Q = Levels of the tests for cognitive impairment	ACE-R 0.47 IQCODE 0.73

2. Paired measures of discrimination:

	Series: IQCODE ≥3.6/5 and ACE-R <73/100	Parallel: IQCODE ≥3.6/5 or ACE-R <73/100
Sensitivity (Se), Specificity (Sp)	0.67, 0.88	0.93, 0.36
PPV, NPV	0.85, 0.72	0.60, 0.83
LR+, LR−	5.38 (large), 0.37 (moderate)	1.45 (slight), 0.19 (large)
CUI+, CUI−	0.57 (adequate), 0.63 (adequate)	0.56 (adequate), 0.30 (very poor)

3. Unitary measures of discrimination:

	Series: IQCODE ≥3.6/5 and ACE-R <73/100	Parallel: IQCODE ≥3.6/5 or ACE-R <73/100
Accuracy	0.77	0.65
Y	0.55	0.29
PSI	0.57	0.43
SUI	1.20 (adequate)	0.86 (poor)

4. Numbers needed:

	Series: IQCODE ≥3.6/5 and ACE-R <73/100	Parallel: IQCODE ≥3.6/5 or ACE-R <73/100
To diagnose (NND)	1.82	3.45
To predict (NNP)	1.75	2.33
To misdiagnose (NNM)	4.35	2.86
Likelihood to be diagnosed or misdiagnosed (NNM/NND, NNM/NNP)	2.39, 2.48	0.83, 1.23
For screening utility (NNSU)	0.83 (adequate)	1.16 (inadequate)

Conclusions:

The pattern of results was similar to that seen with another combination of patient-performance and informant scales (MMSE and IQCODE; Sect. 11.3). LDM, SUI, and NNSU were all adequate for the series combination but inferior in the parallel combination.

11.6 AD8 and 6CIT

Origins:

AD8:

Galvin JE, Roe CM, Powlishta KK, et al. The AD8. A brief informant interview to detect dementia. Neurology. 2005;65:559–64 [5].

6CIT:

Brooke P, Bullock R. Validation of a 6 item cognitive impairment test with a view to primary care usage. Int J Geriatr Psychiatry. 1999;14:936–40 [1].

Contents:

Details on the item content of AD8 and 6CIT may be found in Sects. 7.2 and 4.4 respectively.

Data:

AD8: Quantitative, discrete, ordinal. Score range 8–0, impaired to normal (i.e. negatively scored).

6CIT: Quantitative, discrete, ordinal. Score range 28–0, impaired to normal (i.e. negatively scored).

Pragmatic studies:

Larner AJ. AD8 informant questionnaire for cognitive impairment: pragmatic diagnostic test accuracy study. J Geriatr Psychiatry Neurol. 2015;28:198–202 [11].

Results

For diagnosis of any cognitive impairment:

1. Demographics:

N	169
P = Prevalence of cognitive impairment (= pre-test probability)	0.62
Q = Levels of the tests for cognitive impairment	AD8 0.84, 6CIT 0.69

2. Paired measures of discrimination:

	Series: AD8 ≥2/8 and 6CIT >4/28	Parallel: AD8 ≥2/8 or 6CIT >4/28
Sensitivity (Se), Specificity (Sp)	0.70, 0.13	0.99, 0.59
PPV, NPV	0.57, 0.21	0.80, 0.97
LR+, LR−	0.81 (slight), 2.36 (slight)	2.44 (moderate), 0.02 (very large)
CUI+, CUI−	0.40 (poor), 0.03 (very poor)	0.79 (good), 0.58 (adequate)

3. Unitary measures of discrimination:

	Series: AD8 ≥2/8 and 6CIT >4/28	Parallel: AD8 ≥2/8 or 6CIT >4/28
Accuracy	0.49	0.84
Y	−0.17	0.58
PSI	−0.23	0.77
SUI	0.43 (very poor)	1.37 (good)

4. Numbers needed:

	Series: AD8 ≥2/8 and 6CIT >4/28	Parallel: AD8 ≥2/8 or 6CIT >4/28
To diagnose (NND)	Not calculable	1.72
To predict (NNP)	Not calculable	1.30
To misdiagnose (NNM)	1.96	6.25
Likelihood to be diagnosed or misdiagnosed (NNM/NND, NNM/NNP)	Not calculable	3.63, 4.81
For screening utility (NNSU)	2.33 (inadequate)	0.73 (good)

Conclusions:

These data show some contrasts to those in other combinations reported in this chapter. Although sensitivity, NPV, and LR− were all better in the parallel combination, as anticipated, this also showed the better specificity, PPV, and LR+, parameters usually optimised in the series combination. This pattern differs from that seen with most of the other reported combinations, as noted [12]. The parallel combination also proved better for the unitary measures (LDM, SUI, and NNSU).

11.7   AD8 and MoCA

Origins:

AD8:

Galvin JE, Roe CM, Powlishta KK, et al. The AD8. A brief informant interview to detect dementia. Neurology. 2005;65:559–64 [5].

MoCA:

Nasreddine ZS, Phillips NA, Bédirian V, Charbonneau S, Whitehead V, Collin I, et al. The Montreal Cognitive Assessment, MoCA: a brief screening tool for mild cognitive impairment. J Am Geriatr Soc. 2005;53:695–9 [18].

Contents:

Details on the item content of AD8 and MoCA may be found in Sects. 7.2 and 6.5 respectively.

Data:

AD8: Quantitative, discrete, ordinal. Score range 8–0, impaired to normal (i.e. negatively scored).

MoCA: Quantitative, discrete, ordinal. Score range 0–30, impaired to normal.

Pragmatic studies:

Larner AJ. Does combining an informant questionnaire with patient performance scales improve diagnostic test accuracyfor cognitive impairment? Int J Geriatr Psychiatry. 2017;32:466–7 [12].

Results

For diagnosis of any cognitive impairment:

1. Demographics:

N	46
P = Prevalence of cognitive impairment (= pre-test probability)	0.76
Q = Levels of the tests for cognitive impairment	AD8 0.93, MoCA 0.89

2. Paired measures of discrimination:

	Series: AD8 ≥2/8 and MoCA <26/30	Parallel: AD8 ≥2/8 or MoCA <26/30
Sensitivity (Se), Specificity (Sp)	0.97, 0.45	1.00, 0.18
PPV, NPV	0.85, 0.83	0.80, 1.00
LR+, LR−	1.78 (slight), 0.06 (very large)	1.22 (slight), 0 (very large)
CUI+, CUI−	0.83 (excellent), 0.38 (poor)	0.80 (good), 0.18 (very poor)

3. Unitary measures of discrimination:

	Series: AD8 ≥2/8 and MoCA <26/30	Parallel: AD8 ≥2/8 or MoCA <26/30
Accuracy	0.85	0.80
Y	0.42	0.18
PSI	0.68	0.80
SUI	1.21 (adequate)	0.98 (adequate)

4. Numbers needed:

	Series: AD8 ≥2/8 and MoCA <26/30	Parallel: AD8 ≥2/8 or MoCA <26/30
To diagnose (NND)	2.38	5.56
To predict (NNP)	1.47	1.25
To misdiagnose (NNM)	6.67	5.00

	Series: AD8 ≥2/8 and MoCA <26/30	Parallel: AD8 ≥2/8 or MoCA <26/30
Likelihood to be diag- nosed or misdiagnosed (NNM/NND, NNM/ NNP)	2.80, 4.53	0.90, 4.00
For screening utility (NNSU)	0.83 (adequate)	1.02 (adequate)

Conclusions:

For this combination of patient-performance and informant scales the series combination was evidently better than parallel combination for LDM, SUI, and NNSU, as seen in other similar combinations (Sects. 11.3, 11.4, and 11.5) and unlike the AD8-6CIT combination (Sect. 11.6).

11.8 AD8 and MACE

Origins:

AD8:

Galvin JE, Roe CM, Powlishta KK, et al. The AD8. A brief informant interview to detect dementia. Neurology. 2005;65:559–64 [5].

MACE:

Hsieh S, McGrory S, Leslie F, Dawson K, Ahmed S, Butler CR, et al. The Mini-Addenbrooke's Cognitive Examination: a new assessment tool for dementia. Dement Geriatr Cogn Disord. 2015;39:1–11 [7].

Contents:

Details on the item content of AD8 and MACE may be found in Sects. 7.2 and 5.4 respectively.

Data:

AD8: Quantitative, discrete, ordinal. Score range 8–0, impaired to normal (i.e. negatively scored).

MACE: Quantitative, discrete, ordinal. Score range 0–30, impaired to normal.

Pragmatic studies:

Connon P, Larner AJ. Combining informant (AD8) and patient (MACE) cognitive screening. J Neurol Neurosurg Psychiatry. 2017;88(Suppl1):A20 (PO030) [2].

Larner AJ. Dementia in clinical practice: a neurological perspective. Pragmatic studies in the Cognitive Function Clinic. 3rd ed. London: Springer; 2018. p. 195, 197–8 [13].

Results
For diagnosis of any cognitive impairment:

1. Demographics:

N	67
P = Prevalence of cognitive impairment (= pre-test probability)	0.69
Q = Levels of the tests for cognitive impairment	AD8 0.94, MACE 0.88

2. Paired measures of discrimination:

	Series: AD8 $\geq$2/8 and MACE $\leq$25/30	Parallel: AD8 $\geq$2/8 or MACE $\leq$25/30
Sensitivity (Se), Specificity (Sp)	0.98, 0.43	1.00, 0.10
PPV, NPV	0.79, 0.90	0.71, 1.00
LR+, LR−	1.71 (slight), 0.05 (very large)	1.11 (slight), 0 (very large)
CUI+, CUI−	0.77 (good), 0.39 (poor)	0.71 (good), 0.10 (very poor)

3. Unitary measures of discrimination:

	Series: AD8 $\geq$2/8 and MACE $\leq$25/30	Parallel: AD8 $\geq$2/8 or MACE $\leq$25/30
Accuracy	0.81	0.72
Y	0.41	0.10
PSI	0.69	0.71
SUI	1.16 (adequate)	0.81 (poor)

4. Numbers needed:

	Series: AD8 $\geq$2/8 and MACE $\leq$25/30	Parallel: AD8 $\geq$2/8 or MACE $\leq$25/30
To diagnose (NND)	2.44	10.0
To predict (NNP)	1.45	1.41
To misdiagnose (NNM)	5.26	3.57
Likelihood to be diagnosed or misdiagnosed (NNM/ NND, NNM/NNP)	2.16, 3.63	0.36, 2.54

	Series: AD8 $\geq 2/8$ and MACE $\leq 25/30$	Parallel: AD8 $\geq 2/8$ or MACE $\leq 25/30$
For screening utility (NNSU)	0.86 (adequate)	1.23 (inadequate)

Conclusions:
Unsurprisingly the results were similar to the combination of AD8 and MoCA (Sect. 11.7), with unitary metrics better in the series than in the parallel combination.

References

1. Brooke P, Bullock R. Validation of a 6 item cognitive impairment test with a view to primary care usage. Int J Geriatr Psychiatry. 1999;14:936–40.
2. Connon P, Larner AJ. Combining informant (AD8) and patient (MACE) cognitive screening. J Neurol Neurosurg Psychiatry. 2017;88(Suppl1):A20 (PO030).
3. Cordell CB, Borson S, Boustani M, et al. Medicare Detection of Cognitive Impairment Workgroup. Alzheimer's Association recommendations for operationalizing the detection of cognitive impairment during the Medicare Annual Wellness Visit in a primary care setting. Alzheimers Dement. 2013;9:141–50.
4. Folstein MF, Folstein SE, McHugh PR. Mini-Mental State. A practical method for grading the cognitive state of patients for the clinician. J Psychiatr Res. 1975;12:189–98.
5. Galvin JE, Roe CM, Powlishta KK, et al. The AD8. A brief informant interview to detect dementia. Neurology. 2005;65:559–64.
6. Hancock P, Larner AJ. Diagnostic utility of the Informant Questionnaire on Cognitive Decline in the Elderly (IQCODE) and its combination with the Addenbrooke's Cognitive Examination-Revised (ACE-R) in a memory clinic-based population. Int Psychogeriatr. 2009;21:526–30.
7. Hsieh S, McGrory S, Leslie F, Dawson K, Ahmed S, Butler CR, et al. The Mini-Addenbrooke's Cognitive Examination: a new assessment tool for dementia. Dement Geriatr Cogn Disord. 2015;39:1–11.
8. Jorm AF, Jacomb PA. The Informant Questionnaire on Cognitive Decline in the Elderly (IQCODE): socio-demographic correlates, reliability, validity and some norms. Psychol Med. 1989;19:1015–22.
9. Knafelc R, Lo Giudice D, Harrigan S, et al. The combination of cognitive testing and an informant questionnaire in screening for dementia. Age Ageing. 2003;32:541–7.
10. Larner AJ. Screening utility of the Montreal Cognitive Assessment (MoCA): in place of—or as well as—the MMSE? Int Psychogeriatr. 2012;24:391–6.
11. Larner AJ. AD8 informant questionnaire for cognitive impairment: pragmatic diagnostic test accuracy study. J Geriatr Psychiatry Neurol. 2015;28:198–202.
12. Larner AJ. Does combining an informant questionnaire with patient performance scales improve diagnostic test accuracy for cognitive impairment? Int J Geriatr Psychiatry. 2017;32:466–7.
13. Larner AJ. Dementia in clinical practice: a neurological perspective. Pragmatic studies in the Cognitive Function Clinic. 3rd ed. London: Springer; 2018. p. 195, p. 197–8.

14. Larner AJ. Diagnostic test accuracy studies in dementia. A pragmatic approach. 2nd ed. London: Springer; 2019. p. 81–2, p. 133–6.
15. Mackinnon A, Mulligan R. Combining cognitive testing and informant report to increase accuracy in screening for dementia. Am J Psychiatry. 1988;155:1529–35.
16. Mioshi E, Dawson K, Mitchell J, Arnold R, Hodges JR. The Addenbrooke's Cognitive Examination Revised: a brief cognitive test battery for dementia screening. Int J Geriatr Psychiatry. 2006;21:1078–85.
17. Morley JE, Morris JC, Berg-Weger M, et al. Brain health: the importance of recognizing cognitive impairment: an IAGG consensus conference. J Am Med Dir Assoc. 2015;16:731–9.
18. Nasreddine ZS, Phillips NA, Bédirian V, Charbonneau S, Whitehead V, Collin I, et al. The Montreal Cognitive Assessment, MoCA: a brief screening tool for mild cognitive impairment. J Am Geriatr Soc. 2005;53:695–9.

Chapter 12
Combining Screeners (2): Other Combinations

12.1 Introduction

As for combinations of cognitive screeners reviewed in Chap. 11, other combinations may be undertaken using the same simple logical rules, in series or in parallel.

Patient-based cognitive scales and functional scales may test different constructs, an asymmetry which might afford additional diagnostic information [11]. Scales assessing both cognition and function have been described [5], including Free-Cog (Sect. 6.7).

12.2 Single-Item and Cognitive Screener: SMC Likert Scale and MACE

Origins:
SMC Likert Scale:
Paradise MB, Glozier NS, Naismith SL, Davenport TA, Hickie IB. Subjective memory complaints, vascular risk factors and psychological distress in the middle-aged: a cross-sectional study. BMC Psychiatry. 2011;11:108 [14].

MACE:
Hsieh S, McGrory S, Leslie F, Dawson K, Ahmed S, Butler CR, et al. The Mini-Addenbrooke's Cognitive Examination: a new assessment tool for dementia. Dement Geriatr Cogn Disord. 2015;39:1–11 [6].

Contents:
Details on the item content of SMC Likert scale and MACE may be found in Sects. 2.3 and 5.4 respectively.

© Springer Nature Switzerland AG 2020   135
A. J. Larner, *Manual of Screeners for Dementia*,
https://doi.org/10.1007/978-3-030-41636-2_12

Data:

SMC Likert: Categorical:

- SMC+: those rating their memory as either fair or poor (2 or 1)
- SMC−: those rating their memory as good, very good, or excellent (3, 4, or 5).

MACE: Quantitative, discrete, ordinal. Score range 0–30, impaired to normal.

Pragmatic studies:

Larner AJ. Dementia screening: a different proposal. Future Neurol. 2018;13:177–9 [9].

Results

For diagnosis of no cognitive impairment:

1. Demographics:

N	129
P = Prevalence of cognitive impairment (= pre-test probability)	0.47
Q = Levels of the tests for cognitive impairment	SMC +0.79, MACE 0.76

2. Paired measures of discrimination:

	Series: SMC Likert ≤2 and MACE >25/30	Parallel: SMC Likert ≤2 or MACE >25/30
Sensitivity (Se), Specificity (Sp)	0.29, 0.97	0.94, 0.23
PPV, NPV	0.91, 0.54	0.59, 0.78
LR+, LR−	8.70 (large), 0.73 (slight)	1.23 (slight), 0.25 (moderate)
CUI+, CUI−	0.26 (very poor), 0.52 (adequate)	0.55 (adequate), 0.18 (very poor)

3. Unitary measures of discrimination:

	Series: SMC Likert ≤2 and MACE >25/30	Parallel: SMC Likert ≤2 or MACE >25/30
Accuracy	0.60	0.61
Y	0.26	0.17
PSI	0.45	0.37
SUI	0.78 (poor)	0.73 (poor)

4. Numbers needed:

	Series: SMC Likert ≤ 2 and MACE>25/30	Parallel: SMC Likert ≤ 2 or MACE>25/30
To diagnose (NND)	3.85	5.88
To predict (NNP)	2.22	2.70
To misdiagnose (NNM)	2.50	2.56
Likelihood to be diagnosed or misdiagnosed (NNM/NND, NNM/NNP)	0.65, 1.13	0.43, 0.95
For screening utility (NNSU)	1.28 (inadequate)	1.37 (inadequate)

Conclusions:
As anticipated, series combination improves specificity, PPV, and LR+ at the expense of sensitivity, NPV, and LR−, all of which are better in the parallel combination. The unitary measures and numbers needed slightly favour the series combination, but all are suboptimal.

12.3   Neurological Signs: Triple Test

Origin:
Isik AT, Soysal P, Kaya D, Usarel C. Triple test, a diagnostic observation, can detect cognitive impairment in older adults. Psychogeriatrics. 2018;18:98–105 [7].

Contents:
A combination of the Attended with sign (AW; Sect. 3.2), the Applause sign (AS; Sect. 3.4), and the Head turning sign (HTS; Sect. 3.3) for the diagnosis of cognitive impairment.

Data:
Categorical for all three signs.

Pragmatic studies:
Larner AJ. Response to "Triple test, a diagnostic observation, can detect cognitive impairment in older adults". Psychogeriatrics. 2019;19:407–8 [10].
    Data from:
    Abernethy Holland AJ, Larner AJ. Applause sign: diagnostic utility in a cognitive function clinic. J Neurol Sci. 2013;333:e292 [1].
    Ghadiri-Sani M, Larner AJ. Head turning sign for diagnosis of dementia and mild cognitive impairment: a revalidation. J Neurol Neurosurg Psychiatry. 2013;84:e2 [3].

Results
For diagnosis of any cognitive impairment:

1. Demographics:

N	85
P = Prevalence of cognitive impairment (= pre-test probability)	0.52
Q = Levels of the tests for cognitive impairment	AW 0.68, AS 0.19, HTS 0.48

2. Paired measures of discrimination:

	AW, AS+ and HTS+
Sensitivity (Se), Specificity (Sp)	0.07, 1.00
PPV, NPV	1.00, 0.50
LR+, LR−	∞ (very large), 0.93 (slight)
CUI+, CUI−	0.07 (very poor), 0.50 (adequate)

3. Unitary measures of discrimination:

	AW, AS+ and HTS+
Accuracy	0.52
Y	0.07
PSI	0.50
SUI	0.57 (poor)

4. Numbers needed:

	AW, AS+ and HTS+
To diagnose (NND)	14.3
To predict (NNP)	2.00
To misdiagnose (NNM)	2.08
Likelihood to be diagnosed or misdiagnosed (NNM/NND, NNM/NNP)	0.15, 1.04
For screening utility (NNSU)	1.75 (inadequate)

Conclusions:
The combination of AW and AS+ and HTS+ was rarely encountered in this cohort ($n = 3$; $Q = 0.04$) and had low sensitivity but high specificity, PPV, and LR+. These results are those anticipated with series combination of tests.

The Triple Test has also been examined in combination with the Rapid Cognitive Screening Test [8].

12.4 Functional and Cognitive Screener: IADL Scale and MMSE

Origins:
IADL Scale:
Lawton MP, Brody EM. Assessment of older people: self-maintaining and instrumental activities of daily living. Gerontologist. 1969;9:179–86 [12].
MMSE:
Folstein MF, Folstein SE, McHugh PR. "Mini-Mental State." A practical method for grading the cognitive state of patients for the clinician. J Psychiatr Res. 1975;12:189–98 [2].
NB: Copyright Psychological Assessment Resources.

Contents:
Details on the item content of IADL Scale and MMSE may be found in Sects. 9.2 and 5.2 respectively.

Data:
IADL Scale: Quantitative, discrete, ordinal. Score range = 1–5, higher scores suggest greater impairment.
MMSE: Quantitative, discrete, ordinal. Score range 0–30, impaired to normal.

Pragmatic studies:
Larner AJ. Unpublished. Data from: Hancock P, Larner AJ. The diagnosis of dementia: diagnostic accuracy of an instrument measuring activities of daily living in a clinic-based population. Dement Geriatr Cogn Disord. 2007;23:133–9 [4].

Results
For diagnosis of dementia:

1. Demographics:

N	72
P = Prevalence of dementia (= pre-test probability)	0.54
Q = Levels of the tests for cognitive impairment	IADL 0.67, MMSE 0.35

2. Paired measures of discrimination:

	Series: IADL<14/14 and MMSE<24/30	Parallel: IADL<14/14 or MMSE<24/30
Sensitivity (Se), Specificity (Sp)	0.59, 1.00	0.95, 0.61
PPV, NPV	1.00, 0.67	0.74, 0.91
LR+, LR−	∞ (very large), 0.41 (moderate)	2.41 (moderate), 0.08 (very large)
CUI+, CUI−	0.59 (adequate), 0.67 (good)	0.70 (good), 0.56 (adequate)

3. Unitary measures of discrimination:

	Series: IADL<14/14 and MMSE<24/30	Parallel: IADL<14/14 or MMSE<24/30
Accuracy	0.78	0.79
Y	0.59	0.56
PSI	0.67	0.65
SUI	1.26 (adequate)	1.26 (adequate)

4. Numbers needed:

	Series: IADL<14/14 and MMSE<24/30	Parallel: IADL<14/14 or MMSE<24/30
To diagnose (NND)	1.69	1.79
To predict (NNP)	1.49	1.54
To misdiagnose (NNM)	4.50	4.80
Likelihood to be diagnosed or misdiagnosed (NNM/NND, NNM/NNP)	2.66, 3.02	2.68, 3.12
For screening utility (NNSU)	0.79 (adequate)	0.79 (adequate)

Conclusions:

As anticipated, series combination improves specificity, PPV, and LR+ at the expense of sensitivity, NPV, and LR− which are all better in the parallel combination. The unitary measures and numbers needed show little difference between the series and parallel combinations. These data suggest that combining functional and cognitive screeners may have merit in assessing patients with cognitive impairment.

12.5 Functional and Cognitive Screener: IADL Scale and ACE-R

Origins:
IADL Scale:

Lawton MP, Brody EM. Assessment of older people: self-maintaining and instrumental activities of daily living. Gerontologist. 1969;9:179–86 [12].

ACE-R:

Mioshi E, Dawson K, Mitchell J, Arnold R, Hodges JR. The Addenbrooke's Cognitive Examination Revised: a brief cognitive test battery for dementia screening. Int J Geriatr Psychiatry. 2006;21:1078–85 [13].

Contents:
Details on the item content of IADL Scale and ACE-R may be found in Sects. 9.2 and 6.3 respectively.

Data:
IADL Scale: Quantitative, discrete, ordinal. Score range = 1–5, higher scores suggest greater impairment.

ACE-R: Quantitative, discrete, ordinal. Score range 0–100, impaired to normal.

Pragmatic studies:
Larner AJ, Hancock P. Does combining cognitive and functional scales facilitate the diagnosis of dementia? Int J Geriatr Psychiatry. 2012;27:547–8 [11].

Hancock P, Larner AJ. The diagnosis of dementia: diagnostic accuracy of an instrument measuring activities of daily living in a clinic-based population. Dement Geriatr Cogn Disord. 2007;23:133–9 [4].

Results
For diagnosis of dementia:

1. Demographics:

N	79
P = Prevalence of dementia (= pre-test probability)	0.57
Q = Levels of the tests for cognitive impairment	IADL 0.68, ACE-R 0.47

2. Paired measures of discrimination:

	Series: IADL<14/14 and ACE-R<73/100	Parallel: IADL<14/14 or ACE-R<73/100
Sensitivity (Se), Specificity (Sp)	0.69, 0.94	0.98, 0.59
PPV, NPV	0.94, 0.70	0.76, 0.95
LR+, LR−	11.7 (very large), 0.33 (moderate)	2.37 (moderate), 0.04 (very large)
CUI+, CUI−	0.65 (good), 0.65 (good)	0.74 (good), 0.56 (adequate)

3. Unitary measures of discrimination:

	Series: IADL<14/14 and ACE-R<73/100	Parallel: IADL<14/14 or ACE-R<73/100
Accuracy	0.80	0.81
Y	0.63	0.57
PSI	0.64	0.71
SUI	1.30 (good)	1.30 (good)

4. Numbers needed:

	Series: IADL<14/14 and ACE-R<73/100	Parallel: IADL<14/14 or ACE-R<73/100
To diagnose (NND)	1.59	1.75
To predict (NNP)	1.56	1.41
To misdiagnose (NNM)	5.00	5.26
Likelihood to be diagnosed or misdiagnosed (NNM/NND, NNM/NNP)	3.14, 3.21	3.01, 3.73
For screening utility (NNSU)	0.77 (good)	0.77 (good)

Conclusions:

As anticipated, series combination improves specificity, PPV, and LR+ at the expense of sensitivity, NPV, and LR− which are all better in the parallel combination. The unitary measures and numbers needed show little difference between the series and parallel combinations. Figures are similar to, and perhaps marginally better than, those combining IADL and MMSE (Sect. 12.4). These data suggest that combining functional and cognitive screeners may have merit in assessing patients with cognitive impairment.

References

1. Abernethy Holland AJ, Larner AJ. Applause sign: diagnostic utility in a cognitive function clinic. J Neurol Sci. 2013;333:e292.
2. Folstein MF, Folstein SE, McHugh PR. "Mini-Mental State." A practical method for grading the cognitive state of patients for the clinician. J Psychiatr Res. 1975;12:189–98.
3. Ghadiri-Sani M, Larner AJ. Head turning sign for diagnosis of dementia and mild cognitive impairment: a revalidation. J Neurol Neurosurg Psychiatry. 2013;84:e2.
4. Hancock P, Larner AJ. The diagnosis of dementia: diagnostic accuracy of an instrument measuring activities of daily living in a clinic-based population. Dement Geriatr Cogn Disord. 2007;23:133–9.
5. Heller S, Mendoza Rebolledo C, Rodriguez Blazquez C, Carrasco Chillon L, Perez Munoz A, Rodriguez Perez A, et al. Validation of the multimodal assessment of capacities in severe dementia: a novel cognitive and functional scale for use in severe dementia. J Neurol. 2015;262:1198–208.
6. Hsieh S, McGrory S, Leslie F, Dawson K, Ahmed S, Butler CR, et al. The Mini-Addenbrooke's Cognitive Examination: a new assessment tool for dementia. Dement Geriatr Cogn Disord. 2015;39:1–11.
7. Isik AT, Soysal P, Kaya D, Usarel C. Triple test, a diagnostic observation, can detect cognitive impairment in older adults. Psychogeriatrics. 2018;18:98–105.
8. Koc Okudur S, Dokuzlar O, Kaya D, Soysal P, Isik AT. Triple Test plus Rapid Cognitive Screening Test: a combination of clinical signs and a tool for cognitive assessment in older adults. Diagnostics (Basel). 2019;9:E97.
9. Larner AJ. Dementia screening: a different proposal. Future Neurol. 2018;13:177–9.
10. Larner AJ. Response to "Triple test, a diagnostic observation, can detect cognitive impairment in older adults". Psychogeriatrics. 2019;19:407–8.
11. Larner AJ, Hancock P. Does combining cognitive and functional scales facilitate the diagnosis of dementia? Int J Geriatr Psychiatry. 2012;27:547–8.
12. Lawton MP, Brody EM. Assessment of older people: self-maintaining and instrumental activities of daily living. Gerontologist. 1969;9:179–86.
13. Mioshi E, Dawson K, Mitchell J, Arnold R, Hodges JR. The Addenbrooke's Cognitive Examination Revised: a brief cognitive test battery for dementia screening. Int J Geriatr Psychiatry. 2006;21:1078–85.
14. Paradise MB, Glozier NS, Naismith SL, Davenport TA, Hickie IB. Subjective memory complaints, vascular risk factors and psychological distress in the middle-aged: a cross-sectional study. BMC Psychiatry. 2011;11:108.

Chapter 13
Converting Screeners

13.1 Introduction

Generating data from pragmatic diagnostic test accuracy studies indicates something about test performance, but gives little in the way of comparative data. Test A may perform well, in terms of some or all of the various parameters examined (Fig. 1.1) but that does not necessarily indicate how Test A compares with Test B in a similar clinical situation. For this purpose, head to head studies are ideally required, but these are time consuming and potentially irksome for patients having to complete more than one test. Furthermore, tests need to be administered sequentially in counter-balanced order to avoid bias. Methods to convert test scores may obviate these problems.

In particular, since MMSE scores may be the indicator or determinant for important clinical decisions in cognitively impaired patients, such as the initiation of prescription of cholinesterase inhibitors and/or memantine, converting to MMSE may be relevant.

One method for converting test scores involves the derivation of a conversion table of equivalent scores from equipercentile equating with log-linear smoothing. Examples for MMSE and MoCA are available [9, 10]. Another method is the calculation of linear regression equations.

13.2 Linear Regression Equations

Linear regression equations of the form $y = a + bx$ may be derived to convert test scores.

Here, y, the dependent or outcome variable, is the approximate score of one instrument; x, the independent or explanatory variable, is the score on a different

© Springer Nature Switzerland AG 2020
A. J. Larner, *Manual of Screeners for Dementia*,
https://doi.org/10.1007/978-3-030-41636-2_13

Table 13.1 Regression equations and correlation coefficients of some commonly used cognitive screening instruments (adapted and extended from [7])

Compared CSIs (y vs. x)	N	Regression equation (y = a + bx)	Correlation coefficient (r)
MMSE versus MoCA	147	y = 12.8 + 0.59x	0.85
MMSE versus 6CIT	150	y = 28.1 − 0.44x	−0.73
MMSE versus AD8	125	y = 26.9 − 0.46x	−0.23
MMSE versus MACE	244	y = 12.8 + 0.58x	0.81
MACE versus MoCA	260	y = 4.12 + 0.83x	0.83
MACE versus s-MoCA	260	y = 10.4 + 1.18x	0.79
MACE versus Free-Cog	141	y = −1.42 + 0.97x	0.87
MoCA versus s-MoCA	260	y = 7.53 + 1.43x	0.95

screening instrument with which the first is being compared; and a is the intercept and b the slope or gradient (regression coefficient) of the regression equation. These factors are easily computed (e.g. in Excel) from the datasets of comparative studies.

The datasets of several pragmatic head-to head diagnostic test accuracy studies have been examined in this way (Table 13.1), specifically MMSE versus MoCA [2], MMSE versus 6CIT [1], MMSE versus AD8 [3], MMSE versus MACE [4], MACE versus MoCA [5], MACE versus s-MoCA [6], MACE versus Free-Cog [8], and MoCA versus s-MoCA [6]. Pearson product moment correlation coefficients were also calculated.

As anticipated, since MMSE, MoCA, MACE, s-MoCA and Free-Cog are scored positively and correlate positively their regression coefficients are positive, whereas for 6CIT and AD8, which are negatively scored and correlate negatively with MMSE scores, the slope of the regression line is negative, indicating lower MMSE scores for subjects with higher 6CIT and AD8 scores.

Since MoCA, MACE, 6CIT and AD8 were all more sensitive than MMSE in the base studies, the intercept values of the regression equations were all high, indicating that many correct answers may be achieved on MMSE whilst the other tests remain at floor. MMSE is known to include relatively easy items which are of little value in patient assessment. Greater coincidence of the various test scores occurred around ceiling.

Calculation and application of these regression equations is a relatively simple way to obtain approximate scores when converting between screening instruments. Calculations can be easily done on a mobile phone calculator.

References

1. Abdel-Aziz K, Larner AJ. Six-Item Cognitive Impairment Test (6CIT) for detection of dementia and cognitive impairment. Int Psychogeriatr. 2015;27:991–7.
2. Larner AJ. Screening utility of the Montreal Cognitive Assessment (MoCA): in place of–or as well as—the MMSE? Int Psychogeriatr. 2012;24:391–6.
3. Larner AJ. AD8 informant questionnaire for cognitive impairment: pragmatic diagnostic test accuracy study. J Geriatr Psychiatry Neurol. 2015;28:198–202.
4. Larner AJ. Converting cognitive screening instrument test scores to MMSE scores: regression equations. Int J Geriatr Psychiatry. 2017;32:351–2.
5. Larner AJ. MACE versus MoCA: equivalence or superiority? Pragmatic diagnostic test accuracy study. Int Psychogeriatr. 2017;29:931–7.
6. Larner AJ. Short Montreal Cognitive Assessment: validation and reproducibility. J Geriatr Psychiatry Neurol. 2017;30:104–8.
7. Larner AJ. Dementia in clinical practice: a neurological perspective. Pragmatic studies in the Cognitive Function Clinic. 3rd ed. London: Springer; 2018: 199–200.
8. Larner AJ. Free-Cog: pragmatic test accuracy study and comparison with Mini-Addenbrooke's Cognitive Examination (MACE). Dement Geriatr Cogn Disord. 2019;47:254–63.
9. Roalf DR, Moberg PJ, Xie SX, Wolk DA, Moelter ST, Arnold SE. Comparative accuracies of two common screening instruments for the classification of Alzheimer's disease, mild cognitive impairment and healthy aging. Alzheimers Dement. 2013;9:529–37.
10. van Steenoven I, Aarsland D, Hurtig H, et al. Conversion between mini-mental state examination, Montreal Cognitive Assessment, and Dementia Rating Scale-2 scores in Parkinson's disease. Mov Disord. 2014;29:1809–15.

Chapter 14
Conclusions

14.1 Introduction

One of the purposes of this book has been to present the results of pragmatic screening test accuracy studies in tabular form to allow clinicians to appraise rapidly test performance and hence to inform decisions about potential utility of tests in clinical practice.

Another purpose has been to showcase some new unitary test metrics of potential utility in screening and diagnostic test accuracy studies: the likelihood to be diagnosed or misdiagnosed (LDM), the summary utility index (SUI) and the number needed for screening utility (NNSU; [8]). The development of these metrics stemmed, at least in part, from an awareness of the shortcomings of existing global and unitary test metrics and hence a perception that test accuracy studies were still "underparameterised" with respect to such metrics.

This concluding chapter reviews some existing global test metrics, some of which have been cited throughout this book (see Sect. 1.3.1), as well as the novel unitary measures (Sects. 1.3.4 and 1.3.5) and contrasts them with one another. Whether these latter are adopted may depend on their ease of calculation and perceived utility.

14.2 Existing Global and Unitary Metrics

14.2.1 Accuracy and Net Reclassification Improvement

Accuracy (Acc), also sometimes known as correct classification accuracy, efficiency, effectiveness rate, or posterior probability, is the proportion of correct predictions:

© Springer Nature Switzerland AG 2020
A. J. Larner, *Manual of Screeners for Dementia*,
https://doi.org/10.1007/978-3-030-41636-2_14

$$Acc = (TP + TN)/(TN + FP + FN + TN)$$

Although Acc takes into account all four classes in the 2×2 table (see Fig. 1.2), it treats FN and FP as equally undesirable, which is often not the case in clinical practice.

Acc is the weighted average of sensitivity and specificity, with weights equal to sample prevalence (P):

$$Acc = Sens \times P + Spec \times (1 - P)$$

Hence Acc is not independent of disease prevalence in the test sample.

Net reclassification improvement (NRI) is a parameter which expresses the change in the proportion of individuals correctly classified on the basis of an investigation that is added to the existing diagnostic information. This may be simply calculated as the difference between pre-test probability of diagnosis (or disease prevalence) and posterior probability (or test accuracy; [19]):

$$NRI = Acc - P$$

The dependence of NRI on prevalence means that even a very accurate test may achieve only a small NRI if the diagnosis sought is highly prevalent in the study sample.

14.2.2   Youden Index and Predictive Summary Index

Youden index (Y; [22]), or "informedness" [18], combines information about sensitivity and specificity (as do Likelihood ratios, Sect. 1.3.1):

$$Y = (Sens + Spec) - 1$$
$$= TPR - FPR$$
$$= TP/(TP + FN) - FP/(FP + TN) \qquad (1.4)$$

Thus all four classes in the 2×2 table are taken into account. However, the maximal value of Y arbitrarily assumes disease prevalence to be 50%. Y also treats FN and FP as equally undesirable, which is often not the case in clinical practice.

The predictive summary index (PSI; [15]), or "markedness" [18], combines the positive and negative predictive values:

$$PSI = (PPV + NPV) - 1$$
$$= PPV - FRR$$
$$= TP/(TP + FP) - FN/(FN + TN) \qquad (1.6)$$

Again all four classes in the 2×2 table are taken into account. Like the predictive values, PSI is dependent on disease prevalence.

14.2.3 Diagnostic Odds Ratio

The diagnostic odds ratio (DOR) or cross-product ratio [3, 5] is the ratio of the product of true positives and true negatives and of false negatives and false positives:

$$DOR = TP \times TN/FP \times FN$$

Thus all four classes in the 2×2 table are taken into account. However, DOR gives the most optimistic results by choosing the best quality of a test and ignoring its weaknesses, particularly in populations with very high or very low risk. Ratios become unstable and inflated as the denominator approaches zero, and may be zero or infinite if one of the classes is nil. Like Acc and Y, DOR treats FN and FP as equally undesirable, often not the case in clinical practice. These facts contributed to the decision not to include DOR in the unitary metrics cited in the metrological tables (Fig. 1.1) used throughout this book.

14.2.4 Receiver Operating Characteristic Curve

The receiver operating characteristic (ROC) curve plots false positive rate (FPR = 1 − Spec) on the x axis against Sens or true positive rate (TPR, "hit rate") on the y axis (Fig. 14.1). The area under the curve (AUC ROC) is the probability that a random person with disease has a value of the measurement above the cut-off compared to a random person without disease and hence is a measure of diagnostic accuracy [4, 23].

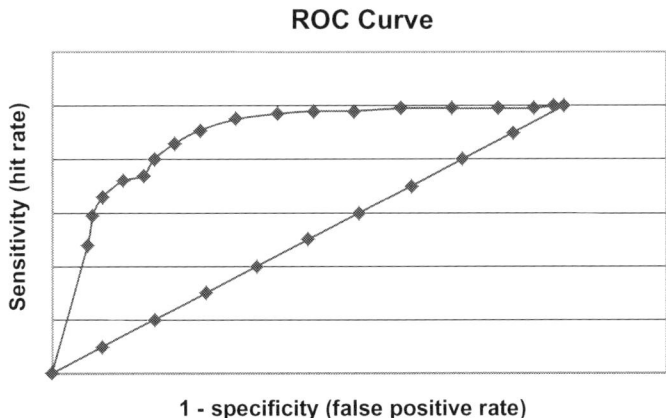

Fig. 14.1 ROC plot of Mini-Addenbrooke's Cognitive Examination for diagnosis of dementia (AUC = 0.89) with chance diagonal (y = x)

The ROC plot ignores TN. It combines test accuracy over a range of thresholds which may be both clinically relevant and clinically nonsensical [16] and thus may be overly optimistic as a global measure of test accuracy [9]. These facts contributed to the decision not to include AUC ROC in the unitary metrics cited in the metrological tables (Fig. 1.1) used throughout this book.

14.2.5   Other Metrics

A number of other metrics are described which might be applicable to the outcomes of screening and diagnostic test accuracy studies but which have been seldom, if ever, used to my knowledge [9]. Some are more familiar in other fields such as machine learning and weather forecasting.

The F measure (F) or F1 score [18] is defined as the harmonic mean of precision (PPV) and recall (Sens):

$$F = 2 \cdot (\text{Sens} \times \text{PPV})/(\text{Sens} + \text{PPV})$$
$$= 2\text{TP}/(2\text{TP} + \text{FP} + \text{FN})$$

Clearly the F measure ignores TN. F measure varies with the chosen test cut-off [10 (Tables 2 and 5), 13].

The threat score (TS) or critical success index is sometimes used in the context of forecasting. TS is defined as the ratio of hits to the sum of hits, false alarms, and misses:

$$\text{TS} = \text{TP}/(\text{TP} + \text{FN} + \text{FP})$$

Clearly TS ignores TN.

Matthews correlation coefficient (MCC) [17] is widely regarded as a very informative score for establishing the quality of a binary classifier:

$$\text{MCC} = (\text{TP} \times \text{TN}) - (\text{FP} \times \text{FN})/\sqrt{(\text{TP} + \text{FP})(\text{TP} + \text{FN})(\text{TN} + \text{FP})(\text{TN} + \text{FN})}$$

MCC takes into account all four classes in the 2×2 table, but its calculation and interpretation may be challenging for clinicians. It was the least optimistic measure of accuracy when examining the outcomes of several test accuracy studies of cognitive screening instruments [9]. MCC varies with the chosen test cut-off [13].

14.3   Novel Unitary Metrics

14.3.1   Likelihood to be Diagnosed or Misdiagnosed (LDM)

The "likelihood to be diagnosed or misdiagnosed" (LDM; [7, 8, 10]) metric was derived as an analogue for test accuracy studies of the "likelihood to be helped or harmed" (LHH) metric used in therapeutic studies [1] (see Sect. 1.3.4).

LDM is based on "number needed" metrics (Sect. 1.3.3), specifically number needed to misdiagnose (NNM = 1/(1 − Acc)), number needed to diagnose (NND = 1/Y), and number needed to predict (NNP = 1/PSI). Hence:

$$
\begin{aligned}
\text{LDM} &= \text{NNM/NND} \\
&= [1/(1 - \text{Acc})]/1/Y \\
&= [1/(\text{FP} + \text{FN})/(\text{TN} + \text{FP} + \text{FN} + \text{TN})]/1/[\text{TP}/(\text{TP} + \text{FN}) \\
&\quad - \text{FP}/(\text{FP} + \text{TN})]
\end{aligned}
\tag{1.9}
$$

or

$$
\begin{aligned}
\text{LDM} &= \text{NNM/NNP} \\
&= [1/(1 - \text{Acc})]/1/\text{PSI} \\
&= 1/(\text{FP} + \text{FN})/(\text{TN} + \text{FP} + \text{FN} + \text{TN})/1/[\text{TP}/(\text{TP} + \text{FP}) \\
&\quad - \text{FN}/(\text{FN} + \text{TN})]
\end{aligned}
\tag{1.10}
$$

Thus LDM takes into account all four classes in the 2×2 table.

Summary "league tables" of LDM values found in pragmatic studies of dementia screeners reported in the previous chapters of this book are shown in Table 14.1.

LDM may have some advantages as a unitary test accuracy metric. Clearly it does not ignore TN, hence is unlike the ROC plot (Sect. 14.2.4), F, and TS (Sect. 14.2.5). Calculation of LDM is relatively straightforward. It has proved applicable to both individual study data [7, 10, 11, 24, 25] and meta-analytic data [20, 24]. LDM also makes explicit the possibility of misdiagnosis when using so-called "diagnostic" tests, an attribute shared with the "number needed to misdiagnose" metric [6].

A number of questions remain concerning the applicability and acceptability of the LDM metric, including but not limited to the following. Firstly, is it possible to categorise LDM values qualitatively, as for likelihood ratios (Table 1.1)? To date, the only distinction made has been between LDM values <1 (undesirable, since more likely to misdiagnose) and >1 (desirable, since more likely to diagnose), with values ≫1 highly desirable [8]. This interpretation mirrors that of likelihood ratios [2]. Low LDM values ($\approx$1) may be indicative of a weakness of tests which it has been suggested might be termed "fragility" [8].

Secondly, should either the NNM/NND or the NNM/NNP metric be the preferred version of LDM, or do both convey unique information? In this context it is of note that NNM/NNP takes into account disease prevalence, since NNP is related to PSI [15], which NND does not.

Thirdly, how do LDM values correlate with other unitary measures? Considering just those (17) screening tests with LDM values for the differentiation of dementia versus no dementia (listed in Table 14.1c), correlation of LDM values with Accuracy was high, likewise for SUI and NNSU (Table 14.2).

Fourthly, how does LDM vary with disease prevalence and with the level of the test, or in other words with values of P and Q (Sect. 1.3.2)? The variation of LDM

Table 14.1 Summary "league tables" of likelihood to be diagnosed or misdiagnosed (LDM = NNM/NND and = NNM/NNP; NNM/NND values prioritised) for: (a) no cognitive impairment; (b) any cognitive impairment; (c) dementia versus no dementia (compare with Table 14.3); (d) mild cognitive impairment (MCI) versus no cognitive impairment

LDM	= NNM/NND	= NNM/NNP
(a)		
AA	0.97	1.02
SMC Likert	0.44	0.65
(b)		
Codex	3.11	3.37
HTS	2.50	2.33
AW	1.02	0.97
Applause	0.72	1.00
CQUIN	0.10	0.10
LMDPP	0.09	0.51
(c)		
ACE-R	7.09	6.91
ACE	4.25	4.25
Codex	3.88	3.29
TYM	3.59	3.71
MMP	3.43	5.01
6CIT	3.30	2.25
Mini-Cog	3.02	2.61
DemTect	2.55	2.64
MACE	2.38	1.31
Free-Cog	2.31	0.93
Applause	1.86	1.66
MMSE	1.56	0.94
IQCODE	0.76	1.00
CBI	0.76	0.71
MoCA	0.54	0.39
AD8	0.12	0.35
s-MoCA	0.08	0.35
(d)		
Mini-Cog	3.09	2.75
s-MoCA	1.83	1.69
MMSE	1.69	1.58
Codex	1.60	2.00
MACE	1.52	1.45
Free-Cog	1.44	1.52
6CIT	1.16	1.06
MMP	1.11	1.53
TYM-MCI	0.97	0.53

Table 14.1   (continued)

LDM	= NNM/NND	= NNM/NNP
MoCA	0.90	0.93
TYM	0.85	0.69
AD8	0.31	0.82

Abbreviations: AA = Attended alone; ACE = Addenbrooke's Cognitive Examination; ACE-R = Addenbrooke's Cognitive Examination-Revised; AW = Attended with; CBI = Cambridge Behavioural Inventory; LMDPP = *La maladie du petit papier*; HTS = Head turning sign; IQCODE = Informant Questionnaire on Cognitive Decline in the Elderly; MACE = Mini-Addenbrooke's Cognitive Examination; MMSE = Mini-Mental State Examination; MMP = Mini-Mental Parkinson; MoCA = Montreal Cognitive Assessment; 6CIT = Six-Item Cognitive Impairment Test; s-MoCA = Short Montreal Cognitive Assessment; TYM = Test Your Memory test

Table 14.2 Correlations between unitary test metric values for 17 different screening tests for diagnosis of dementia versus no dementia listed in Table 14.1c)

	r
LDM = NNM/NND:	
Accuracy	0.83
NNM/NNP	0.93
SUI	0.93
NNSU	−0.77
LDM = NNM/NNP:	
Accuracy	0.77
SUI	0.87
NNSU	−0.68
SUI:	
Accuracy	0.96
NNSU	−0.93
NNSU:	
Accuracy	−0.98

values with P may be looked at in two ways: by calculation at fixed values of P, and empirically.

LDM values may be calculated using the methods for determining values of PPV and NPV at fixed values of P, as per Eqs. 1.1 and 1.2:

$$PPV = Sens \times P/(Sens \times P) + [(1 - Spec) \times P']$$ (1.1)

$$NPV = Spec \times P'/[Spec \times P'][(1 - Sens) \times P]$$ (1.2)

Hence values for PSI and NNP may be calculated as per Eqs. 1.6 and 1.7:

$$PSI = (PPV + NPV) - 1$$ (1.6)

$$NNP = 1/PSI$$ (1.7)

Acc may be calculated at fixed values of P as per Eq. 1.3:

$$Acc = Sens \times P + Spec \times P'$$ (1.3)

Hence NNM may be calculated as per Eq. 1.8:

$$NNM = 1/Inacc = 1/(1 - Acc) \qquad (1.8)$$

The values of Sens and Spec for these calculations are fixed by the chosen test cut-off. The cut-off value may vary according to the method chosen to determine the dichotomisation point (Sect. 1.3.1). Using data from a previously reported test accuracy study of Mini-Addenbrooke's Cognitive Examination (MACE; score range 0–30; [10]), LDM values have been calculated at cut-offs determined by maximal Youden index ($\leq$20/30) and maximal correct classification accuracy ($\leq$14/30), as shown in Fig. 1.3. These choices also determine Y and hence NND for each of these cut-offs. From NNM, NNP, and fixed NND, values of LDM = NNM/NND and NNM/NNP may be calculated (Table 14.3) and plotted (Figs. 14.2 and 14.3). Note that for these purposes, absolute ("raw") values of all the number needed metrics have been used, they have not been rounded up to the next highest positive integer, as required for clinical utility (Sect. 1.3.3).

Clearly these plots show curves of different shape dependent on the chosen cut-off.

One obvious limitation of the "league table" of LDM values (Table 14.1) is that the results are true only for the groups investigated in each individual pragmatic test accuracy study, each of which differs in exact case mix and hence prevalence of the diagnosis of interest, such as dementia or MCI. Hence the results are not truly comparable. One way around this would be to scale for an arbitrarily fixed prevalence, P, and use Eqs. 1.1, 1.2 and 1.3 to calculate PPV, NPV and Acc respectively, and hence NNP and NNM so that a value of LDM for a fixed value of P common to all studies may be calculated. A scaled "league table" of LDM values for dementia versus no dementia at P = 0.2 is shown in Table 14.4, for comparison with Table 14.1c). Such scaled results may be more generalizable.

The variation of LDM values with P may also be examined empirically [14]. In a study looking at MACE performance in patient subgroups determined by age, P is higher in the older age groups (age$\geq$ 65 years and $\geq$75 years) compared to the whole cohort (median age 60 years). In other words, these subgroups are enriched for the target disorder [21]. These empirical data (Table 14.5) show NNM/NND falls with increasing prevalence, whereas NNM/NNP rises. This pattern coincides with the values calculated using the maximal accuracy cut-off (Fig. 14.3) but not when using the maximal Youden index cut-off (Fig. 14.2). Further exploration of these discrepancies in studies of other screening tests administered in other settings may be worthwhile.

The variation of LDM values with Q might, as for P, be looked at in two ways, by calculation at fixed values of Q [12], and empirically. However, it is most straightforward to do this analysis empirically by looking at test performance at different test cut-offs, as illustrated using data from the MACE study [10 (Table 3), 12] (Fig. 14.4).

Evidently LDM varies with test cut-off. The maxima for both NNM/NND and NNM/NNP appear to coincide with the maximal test accuracy cut-off (compare Fig. 14.4 with Fig. 1.3). Again this will need to be investigated in datasets of further studies.

Table 14.3 (a) LDM values of MACE for dementia diagnosis at various prevalence levels at fixed Sens and Spec with cut-off determined by maximal Youden index (0.619) and hence fixed NND (=1.616). See Fig. 14.2. (b) LDM values of MACE for dementia diagnosis at various prevalence levels at fixed Sens and Spec with cut-off determined by maximal accuracy (0.867) and hence fixed NND (=1.980). See Fig. 14.3

P, P'	PPV, NPV	PSI	NNP	Acc, Inacc	NNM	LDM=NNM/NND	LDM=NNM/NNP
(a)							
0.1, 0.9	0.257, 0.986	0.243	4.11	0.727, 0.272	3.67	2.70	0.89
0.2, 0.8	0.437, 0.970	0.407	2.45	0.748, 0.252	3.97	2.45	1.62
0.3, 0.7	0.571, 0.949	0.521	1.92	0.768, 0.232	4.32	2.67	2.25
0.4, 0.6	0.675, 0.924	0.598	1.67	0.789, 0.211	4.74	2.93	2.83
0.5, 0.5	0.757, 0.890	0.646	1.55	0.809, 0.191	5.25	3.25	3.39
0.6, 0.4	0.824, 0.843	0.667	1.50	0.830, 0.170	5.88	3.64	3.92
0.7, 0.3	0.879, 0.775	0.654	1.53	0.851, 0.149	6.69	4.14	4.38
0.8, 0.2	0.926, 0.668	0.594	1.68	0.871, 0.129	7.76	4.80	4.61
0.9, 0.1	0.966, 0.472	0.438	2.28	0.892, 0.108	9.24	5.72	4.04
(b)							
0.1, 0.9	0.441, 0.952	0.394	2.54	0.884, 0.116	8.65	4.37	3.40
0.2, 0.8	0.640, 0.899	0.539	1.86	0.851, 0.149	6.73	3.40	3.63
0.3, 0.7	0.753, 0.838	0.591	1.69	0.818, 0.182	5.51	2.78	3.26
0.4, 0.6	0.826, 0.769	0.595	1.68	0.785, 0.215	4.66	2.35	2.77
0.5, 0.5	0.877, 0.690	0.567	1.76	0.753, 0.247	4.04	2.04	2.29
0.6, 0.4	0.914, 0.597	0.512	1.95	0.720, 0.280	3.57	1.80	1.82
0.7, 0.3	0.943, 0.488	0.431	2.32	0.687, 0.313	3.19	1.61	1.38
0.8, 0.2	0.966, 0.357	0.323	3.09	0.654, 0.346	2.89	1.46	0.93
0.9, 0.1	0.985, 0.198	0.183	5.47	0.621, 0.379	2.64	1.33	0.48

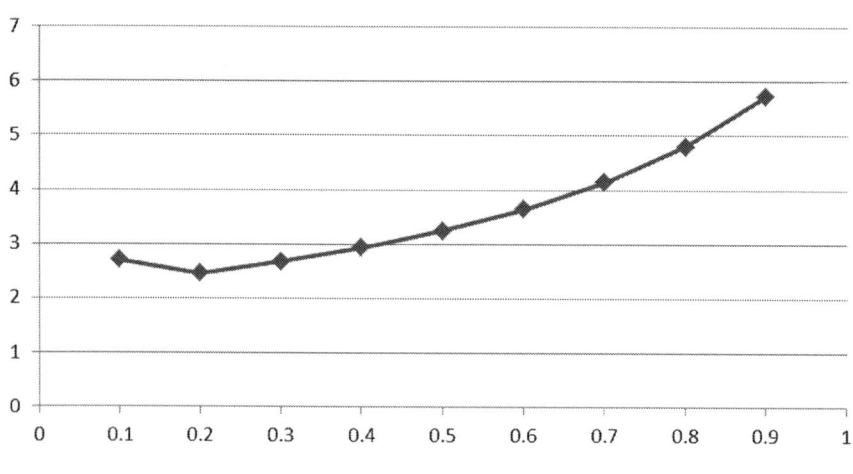

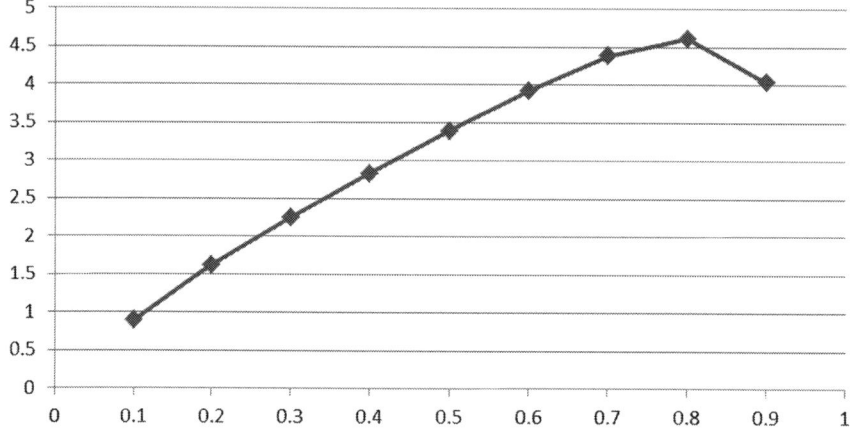

Fig. 14.2 Plot of LDM values (y axis) of MACE for dementia diagnosis versus prevalence (x axis) for maximal Youden index cut-off (data from Table 14.3a)

14.3.2   Summary Utility Index (SUI) and its Reciprocal (NNSU)

The summary utility index (SUI) and the number needed for screening utility (NNSU) metrics were initially conceived as analogues of Y and NND although their eventual empirical derivation differed from these [8] (see Sect. 1.3.5).

$$SUI = CUI+ + \ CUI-$$
$$= (Sens \ \times \ PPV) + (Spec \ \times \ NPV)$$
$$= \left[TP^2/(TP + FN)(TP + FP)\right] + \left[TN^2/(TN + FP)(TN + FN)\right] \quad (1.11)$$

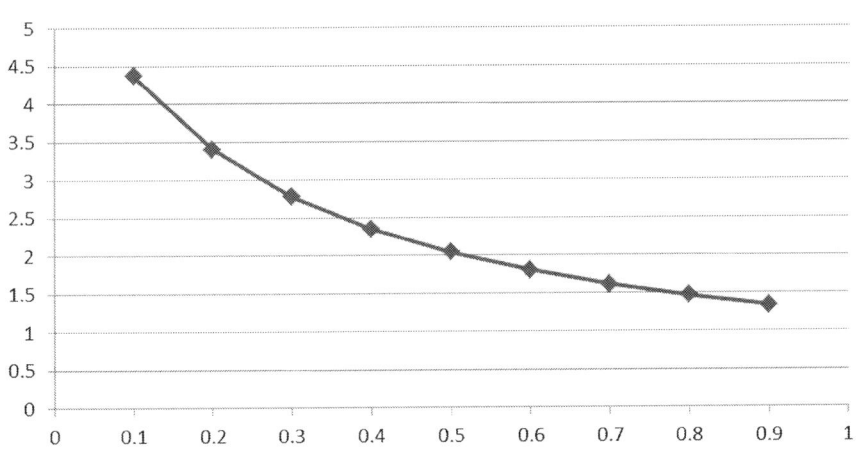

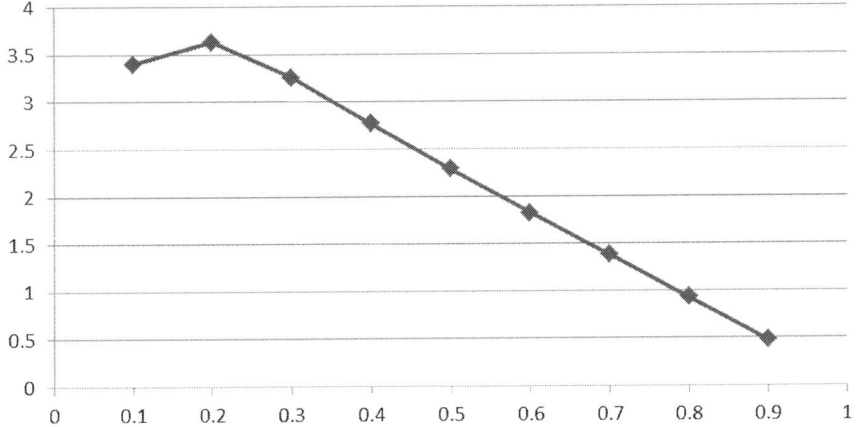

Fig. 14.3 Plot of LDM values (y axis) of MACE for dementia diagnosis versus prevalence (x axis) for maximal accuracy cut-off (data from Table 14.3b)

$$\begin{aligned} NNSU &= 1/SUI \\ &= 1/(CUI+ + CUI-) \\ &= 1/(Sens \times PPV) + (Spec \times NPV) \\ &= 1/\left[TP^2/(TP + FN)(TP + FP)\right] + \left[TN^2/(TN + FP)(TN + FN)\right] (1.12) \end{aligned}$$

Thus both SUI and NNSU take into account all four classes in the 2×2 table.

Table 14.4 Summary "league tables" of calculated likelihood to be diagnosed or misdiagnosed (LDM = NNM/NNP) at fixed value of P (= 0.2) for diagnosis of dementia versus no dementia. Compare with Table 14.1c) column 2

LDM	= NNM/NNP
ACE-R	6.87
MMP	5.72
TYM	3.55
ACE	3.09
Codex	2.80
6CIT	2.31
Mini-Cog	1.77
Applause	1.67
Free-Cog	1.63
MACE	1.62
DemTect	1.47
MMSE	1.02
CBI	0.75
MoCA	0.48
IQCODE	0.35
AD8	0.23
s-MoCA	0.19

Abbreviations: ACE = Addenbrooke's Cognitive Examination; ACE-R = Addenbrooke's Cognitive Examination-Revised; CBI = Cambridge Behavioural Inventory; IQCODE = Informant Questionnaire on Cognitive Decline in the Elderly; MACE = Mini-Addenbrooke's Cognitive Examination; MMSE = Mini-Mental State Examination; MMP = Mini-Mental Parkinson; MoCA = Montreal Cognitive Assessment; 6CIT = Six-Item Cognitive Impairment Test; s-MoCA = Short Montreal Cognitive Assessment; TYM = Test Your Memory test

Table 14.5 LDM values of MACE for diagnosis of dementia versus no dementia using MACE cut-off ≤25/30 in whole cohort versus cohorts of older patients (aged ≥65 and ≥75 years)

	Whole cohort	Older patients aged ≥65 years	Older patients aged ≥75 years
N	755	287	119
Dementia prevalence (P)	0.151	0.272	0.387
Likelihood to be diagnosed or misdiagnosed (LDM):			
= NNM/NND	0.53	0.39	0.09
= NNM/NNP	0.34	0.56	0.69

Summary "league tables" of SUI and NNSU values found in pragmatic studies of dementia screeners reported in previous chapters of this book are shown in Table 14.6.

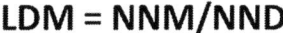

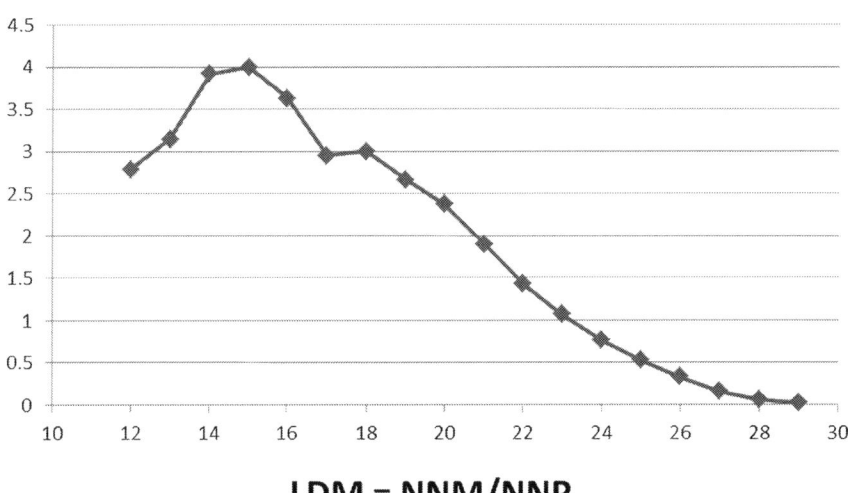

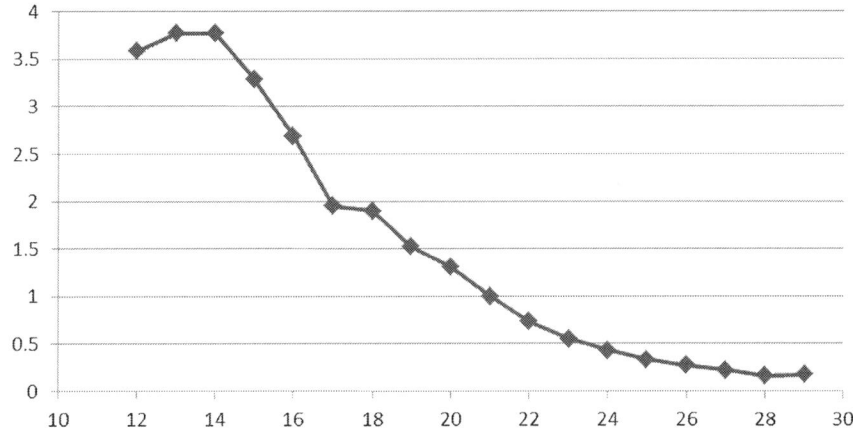

Fig. 14.4 Plot of LDM values (y axis) versus MACE cut-off (x-axis; data from Larner [10])

SUI and NNSU may have some advantages as unitary test accuracy metrics. All cells of the 2 × 2 table are taken into account. The values are easily classified qualitatively, based on the classification of clinical utility indexes (Tables 1.3 and 1.4).

As for LDM, a number of questions remain concerning the applicability and acceptability of SUI and NNSU metrics. How these measures correlate with other unitary measures is shown in Table 14.2.

How the values of SUI and NNSU vary with disease prevalence and with test cut-off, that is with values of P and Q (Sect. 1.3.2), is of interest. This may be

Table 14.6 Summary "league tables" of summary utility index (SUI) and number needed for screening utility (NNSU) for: (a) no cognitive impairment; (b) any cognitive impairment; (c) dementia versus no dementia; (d) mild cognitive impairment (MCI) versus no cognitive impairment

	SUI	NNSU
(a)		
AA	0.86	1.16
SMC Likert	0.72	1.39
(b)		
Codex	1.30	0.77
HTS	1.20	0.83
AW	0.86	1.16
Applause	0.85	1.18
CQUIN	0.54	1.85
LMDPP	0.48	2.08
(c)		
ACE-R	1.57	0.64
ACE	1.42	0.70
TYM	1.32	0.76
Codex	1.30	0.77
MMP	1.26	0.79
DemTect	1.23	0.81
Mini-Cog	1.19	0.84
6CIT	1.18	0.85
MACE	1.03	0.97
Applause	1.00	1.00
Free-Cog	0.94	1.06
MMSE	0.90	1.11
IQCODE	0.84	1.19
CBI	0.79	1.27
MoCA	0.53	1.89
s-MoCA	0.43	2.33
AD8	0.40	2.50
(d)		
Mini-Cog	1.18	0.85
s-MoCA	1.07	0.93
MMSE	1.03	0.97
Free-Cog=	1.00	1.00
MACE=	1.00	1.00
Codex	0.99	1.01
MMP	0.92	1.09
6CIT	0.91	1.10

Table 14.6 (continued)

	SUI	NNSU
MoCA	0.83	1.20
TYM	0.79	1.27
TYM-MCI	0.78	1.28
AD8	0.64	1.56

Abbreviations: AA = Attended alone; ACE = Addenbrooke's Cognitive Examination; ACE-R = Addenbrooke's Cognitive Examination-Revised; AW = Attended with; CBI = Cambridge Behavioural Inventory; LMDPP = *La maladie du petit papier*; HTS = Head turning sign; IQCODE = Informant Questionnaire on Cognitive Decline in the Elderly; MACE = Mini-Addenbrooke's Cognitive Examination; MMSE = Mini-Mental State Examination; MMP = Mini-Mental Parkinson; MoCA = Montreal Cognitive Assessment; 6CIT = Six-Item Cognitive Impairment Test; s-MoCA = Short Montreal Cognitive Assessment; TYM = Test Your Memory test

Table 14.7 a SUI and NNSU values of MACE for dementia diagnosis at various prevalence levels at fixed Sens and Spec with cut-off determined by maximal Youden index (0.619) and hence fixed NND (= 1.616). See Fig. 14.5. b: SUI and NNSU values of MACE for dementia diagnosis at various prevalence levels at fixed Sens and Spec with cut-off determined by maximal accuracy (0.867) and hence fixed NND (= 1.980). See Fig. 14.6

P, P′	CUI+, CUI−	SUI	NNSU
(a)			
0.1, 0.9	0.234 (very poor), 0.697 (good)	0.931 (poor)	1.074 (inadequate)
0.2, 0.8	0.399 (poor), 0.685 (good)	1.085 (adequate)	0.922 (adequate)
0.3, 0.7	0.521 (adequate), 0.671 (good)	1.192 (adequate)	0.839 (adequate)
0.4, 0.6	0.615 (adequate), 0.653 (good)	1.268 (adequate)	0.789 (adequate)
0.5, 0.5	0.690 (good), 0.629 (adequate)	1.319 (good)	0.758 (good)
0.6, 0.4	0.751 (good), 0.596 (adequate)	1.347 (good)	0.742 (good)
0.7, 0.3	0.802 (good), 0.548 (adequate)	1.350 (good)	0.741 (good)
0.8, 0.2	0.844 (excellent), 0.472 (poor)	1.317 (good)	0.759 (good)
0.9, 0.1	0.881 (excellent), 0.334 (very poor)	1.214 (adequate)	0.823 (adequate)
(b)			
0.1, 0.9	0.259 (very poor), 0.874 (excellent)	1.133 (adequate)	0.883 (adequate)
0.2, 0.8	0.376 (poor), 0.825 (excellent)	1.201 (adequate)	0.833 (adequate)
0.3, 0.7	0.442 (poor), 0.769 (good)	1.212 (adequate)	0.825 (adequate)
0.4, 0.6	0.485 (poor), 0.706 (good)	1.191 (adequate)	0.840 (adequate)
0.5, 0.5	0.515 (adequate), 0.633 (adequate)	1.148 (adequate)	0.871 (adequate)
0.6, 0.4	0.537 (adequate), 0.548 (adequate)	1.085 (adequate)	0.921 (adequate)
0.7, 0.3	0.554 (adequate), 0.448 (poor)	1.002 (adequate)	0.998 (adequate)
0.8, 0.2	0.568 (adequate), 0.328 (very poor)	0.896 (poor)	1.117 (inadequate)
0.9, 0.1	0.579 (adequate), 0.182 (very poor)	0.761 (poor)	1.315 (inadequate)

examined both by calculation and empirically. By calculation, using the fixed values of Sens and Spec and the calculated values of PPV and NPV (Eqs. 1.1 and 1.2) it is possible to calculate CUI+ (=Sens × PPV) and CUI− (=Spec × NPV) and hence SUI and NNSU as per Eqs. 1.11 and 1.12.

Using data from a previously reported test accuracy study of MACE (score range 0–30; [10, 13]), at cut-offs determined by maximal Youden index ($\leq$20/30) and maximal correct classification accuracy ($\leq$14/30), SUI and NNSU values have been calculated (Table 14.7) and plotted (Figs. 14.5 and 14.6). Note that for these purposes, absolute ("raw") values of NNSU have been used, they have not been rounded up to the next highest positive integer, as required for clinical meaning (Sect. 1.3.3).

Clearly these plots show curves of different shape dependent on the chosen cut-off.

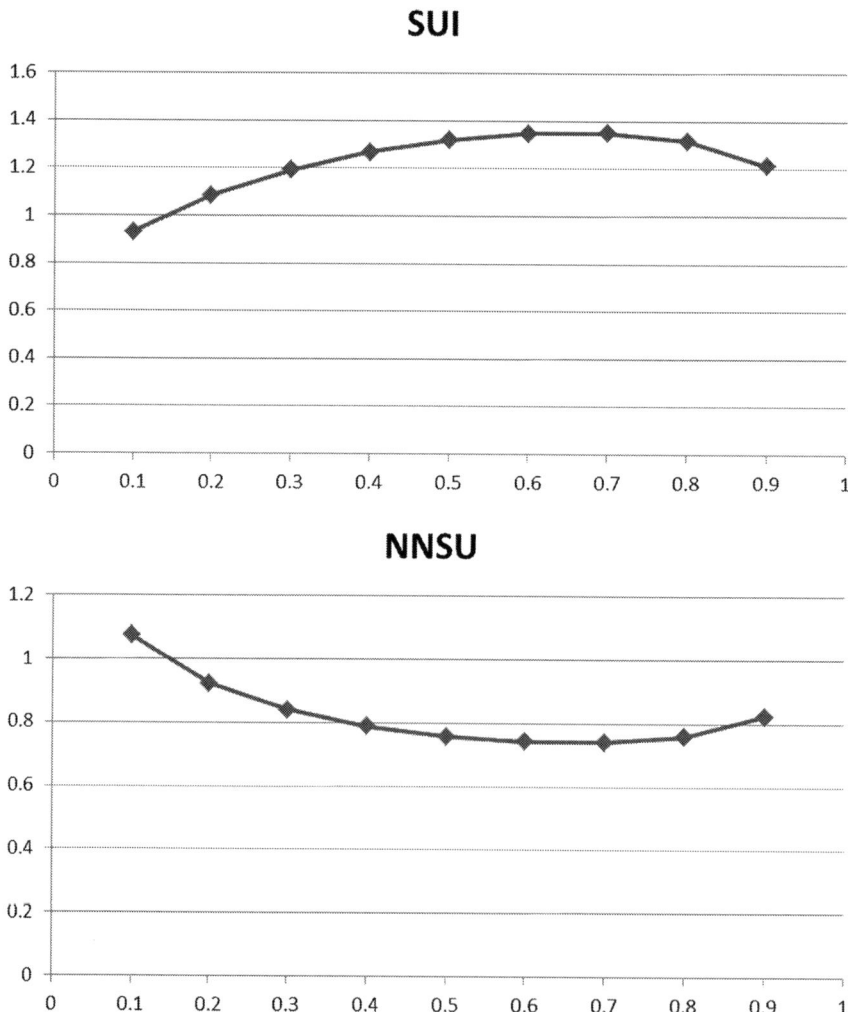

Fig. 14.5 Plot of SUI and NNSU values (y axis) of MACE for dementia diagnosis versus prevalence (x axis) for maximal Youden index cut-off (data from Table 14.7a)

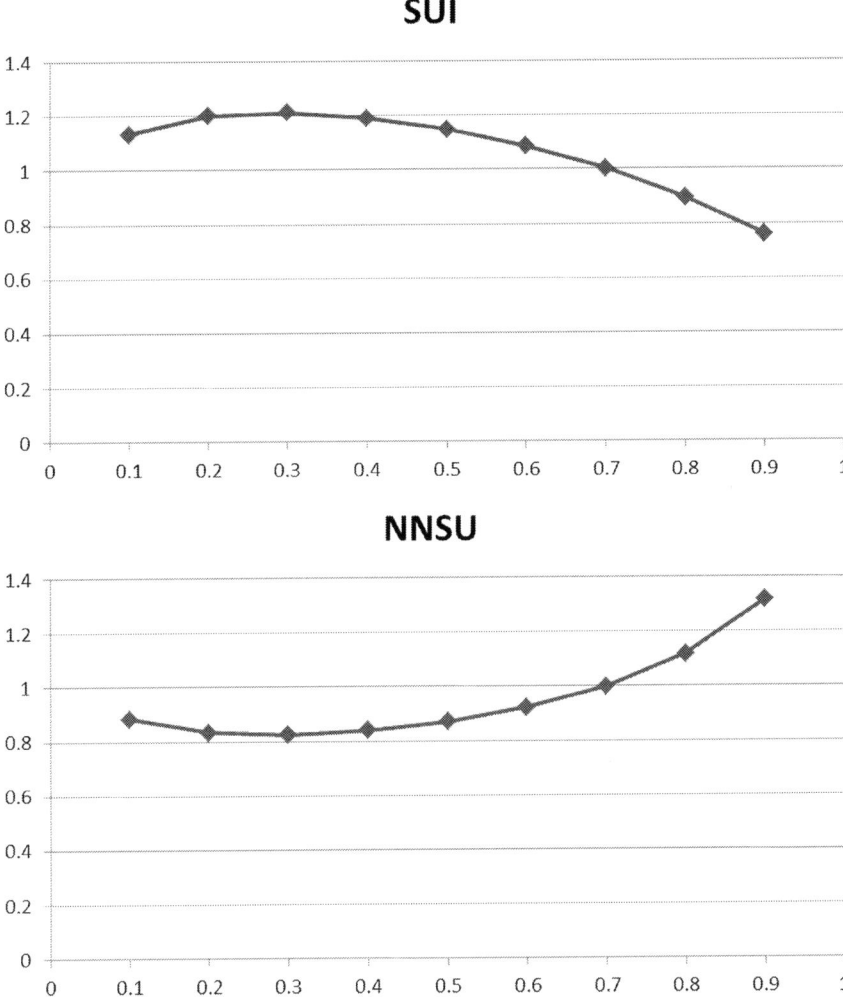

Fig. 14.6 Plot of SUI and NNSU values (y axis) of MACE for dementia diagnosis versus prevalence (x axis) for maximal accuracy cut-off (data from Table 14.7b)

Table 14.8 SUI and NNSU values for diagnosis of dementia versus no dementia using MACE cut-off $\leq$25/30 in whole cohort versus cohorts of older patients (aged $\geq$65 and $\geq$75 years)

	Whole cohort	Older patients aged $\geq$65 years	Older patients aged $\geq$75 years
N	755	287	119
Dementia prevalence (P)	0.151	0.272	0.387
Summary Utility Index (SUI = CUI+ + CUI−)	0.51 (very poor)	0.54 (very poor)	0.45 (very poor)
Number needed for screening utility (NNSU = 1/SUI)	1.94 (inadequate)	1.85 (inadequate)	2.22 (inadequate)

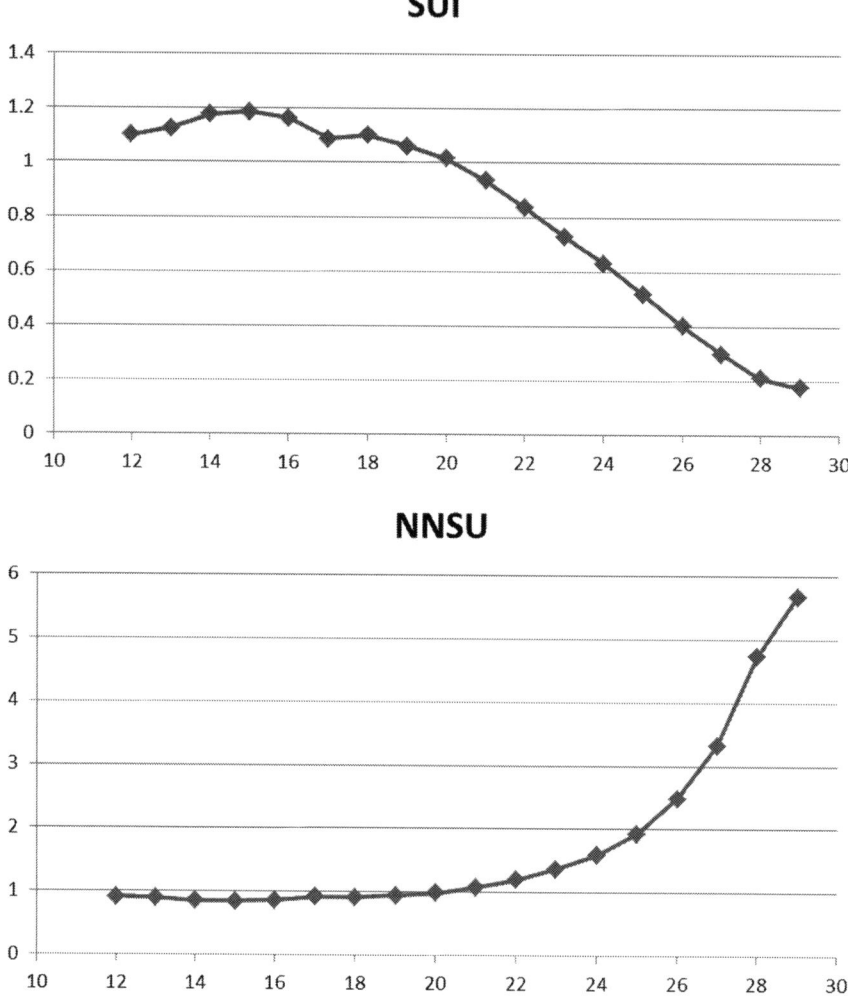

Fig. 14.7 Plot of SUI and NNSU values (y axis) versus MACE cut-off (x-axis; data from Larner [10])

The variation of SUI and NNSU values with P has also been examined empirically in patient subgroups determined by age [14] (see Table 14.8).

These empirical data suggest SUI and NNSU show little change with increasing prevalence. This pattern appears to coincide with the values calculated using both the maximal Youden index cut-off (Fig. 14.5) and the maximal accuracy cut-off (Fig. 14.6). Obviously further exploration of these observations in studies of other screening tests administered in other settings is required.

The variation of SUI and NNSU values with Q is most straightforwardly examined by looking at test performance at different cut-offs, as illustrated using data from the MACE study [10 (Tables 2, 3, 5 and 6), 13] (Fig. 14.7).

Evidently SUI and NNSU vary with test cut-off. The maximum for SUI appears to coincide with the maximal test accuracy cut-off (compare Figs. 14.7 and 1.3). Again this will need to be investigated in further study datasets.

14.4 Summary

The novel unitary test metrics, LDM, SUI, and NNSU, may have some advantages over existing unitary metrics. However, if they are to be adopted, a broadening of clinician literacy will be required, although the underlying concepts and calculations are simple, and the outcome measures may be deemed intuitive and easily communicable to other clinicians and to patients. Like the existing metrics they are potentially applicable to any screening or diagnostic test in any area of medical or surgical practice.

Evidently this is a work in progress. Time and usage will be the final arbiters of whether these heuristics become aids to practice and elements of the empirical science of screening test accuracy studies.

References

1. Citrome L, Ketter TA. When does a difference make a difference? Interpretation of number needed to treat, number needed to harm, and likelihood to be helped or harmed. Int J Clin Pract. 2013;67:407–11.
2. Deeks JJ, Altman DG. Diagnostic tests 4: likelihood ratios. BMJ. 2004;329:168–9.
3. Edwards AWF. The measure of association in a 2x2 table. J R Stat Soc Ser A. 1963;126:109–14.
4. Fawcett T. An introduction to ROC analysis. Pattern Recognit Lett. 2006;27:861–74.
5. Glas AS, Lijmer JG, Prins MH, Bonsel GJ, Bossuyt PM. The diagnostic odds ratio: a single indicator of test performance. J Clin Epidemiol. 2003;56:1129–35.
6. Habibzadeh F, Yadollahie M. Number needed to misdiagnose: a measure of diagnostic test effectiveness. Epidemiology. 2013;24:170.
7. Larner AJ. Number needed to diagnose, predict, or misdiagnose: useful metrics for non-canonical signs of cognitive status? Dement Geriatr Cogn Dis Extra. 2018;8:321–7.
8. Larner AJ. New unitary metrics for dementia test accuracy studies. Prog Neurol Psychiatry. 2019a;23(3):21–5.
9. Larner AJ. What is test accuracy? Comparing unitary accuracy metrics for cognitive screening instruments. Neurodegener Dis Manag. 2019b;9:277–81.
10. Larner AJ. MACE for diagnosis of dementia and MCI: examining cut-offs and predictive values. Diagnostics (Basel). 2019c;9:E51.
11. Larner AJ. Evaluating cognitive screening instruments with the "likelihood to be diagnosed or misdiagnosed" measure. Int J Clin Pract. 2019d;73:e13265.
12. Larner AJ. Applying Kraemer's Q (positive sign rate): some implications for diagnostic test accuracy study results. Dement Geriatr Cogn Dis Extra. 2019e;9:389–96.

13. Larner AJ. Defining "optimal" test cut-off using global test metrics: evidence from a cognitive screening instrument. 2020a;submitted.
14. Larner AJ. Mini-Addenbrooke's Cognitive Examination (MACE): a useful cognitive screening instrument in older people? Can Geriatr J. 2020b;23:in press.
15. Linn S, Grunau PD. New patient-oriented summary measure of net total gain in certainty for dichotomous diagnostic tests. Epidemiol Perspect Innov. 2006;3:11.
16. Mallett S, Halligan S, Thompson M, Collins GS, Altman DG. Interpreting diagnostic accuracy studies for patient care. BMJ. 2012;345:e3999.
17. Matthews BW. Comparison of the predicted and observed secondary structure of T4 phage lysozyme. Biochem Biophys Acta. 1975;405:442–51.
18. Powers DMW. Evaluation: from precision, recall and F-measure to ROC, informedness, markedness and correlation. J Machine Learning Technologies. 2011;2:37–63.
19. Richard E, Schmand BA, Eikelenboom P, Van Gool WA, The Alzheimer's Disease Neuroimaging Initiative. MRI and cerebrospinal fluid biomarkers for predicting progression to Alzheimer's disease in patients with mild cognitive impairment: a diagnostic accuracy study. BMJ Open. 2013;3:e002541.
20. Williamson JC, Larner AJ. "Likelihood to be diagnosed or misdiagnosed": application to meta-analytic data for cognitive screening instruments. Neurodegener Dis Manag. 2019;9:91–5.
21. Wojtowicz A, Larner AJ. Diagnostic test accuracy of cognitive screeners in older people. Prog Neurol Psychiatry. 2017;21(1):17–21.
22. Youden WJ. Index for rating diagnostic tests. Cancer. 1950;3:32–5.
23. Youngstrom EA. A primer on receiver operating characteristic analysis and diagnostic efficiency statistics for pediatric psychology: we are ready to ROC. J Pediatr Psychol. 2014;39:204–21.
24. Ziso B, Larner AJ. AD8: Likelihood to diagnose or misdiagnose. J Neurol Neurosurg Psychiatry. 2019a;90:A20. https://jnnp.bmj.com/content/90/12/A20.1.
25. Ziso B, Larner AJ. Codex (cognitive disorders examination) decision tree modified for the detection of dementia and MCI. Diagnostics (Basel). 2019;9:E58.

Index

A

Accuracy (Acc), 2–4, 6–12, 14, 20, 22, 26, 27,
    29, 31–34, 36, 40, 41, 44, 45, 47, 48,
    53, 55–57, 59, 61, 62, 64, 65, 67, 71,
    73–75, 77–81, 83, 84, 91, 93, 95,
    100, 102–104, 108–110, 115, 116,
    121, 123–125, 127, 128, 130, 132,
    136, 138–142, 145, 146, 149–153,
    155–157, 159, 161, 163–167

ACE-III, ACEmobile, 58, 73, 75, 76

AD8. *See* Ascertain Dementia 8

Addenbrooke's Cognitive Examination (ACE),
    8, 54, 60, 71–73, 76, 154, 155, 160,
    162, 163

Addenbrooke's Cognitive
    Examination-Revised (ACE-R), 8,
    54, 58, 60, 74–76, 93, 94, 109, 122,
    125–127, 141, 142, 154, 155, 160,
    162, 163

"And" rule, 119

Applause sign, 11, 14, 32, 34, 35, 137

Area Under the Receiver Operating
    Characteristic Curve (AUC ROC),
    3, 71, 151, 152

Ascertain Dementia 8 (AD8), 11, 14, 54, 90,
    92, 124, 125, 127–133, 146, 154,
    155, 160, 162, 163

Attended Alone (AA) sign, 25, 26, 28, 29

Attended With (AW) sign, 26, 28, 30, 137

AW2+ sign, 30

C

Cambridge Behavioural Inventory (CBI), 95,
    96, 154, 155, 160, 162, 163

Clinical Utility Indexes (CUI+, CUI−), 5, 7,
    8, 11–14, 20, 22, 26, 27, 29, 31, 33,
    34, 36, 40, 41, 44, 45, 47, 48, 52,
    53, 56–59, 61, 62, 64, 65, 67, 72,
    75, 78, 80, 81, 83, 84, 90, 91, 93,
    95, 100, 102, 104, 108, 110, 115,
    116, 120, 122, 124, 126, 128, 130,
    132, 136, 138, 140, 142, 158, 161,
    163, 165

Cognitive disorders examination (Codex),
    11, 39, 40, 42, 43, 46, 154, 160,
    162

Combining screeners, 89, 143

Confusion matrix/table, 3

Cornell Scale for Depression in Dementia
    (CSDD), 89, 103, 104

Correct classification accuracy. *See* accuracy

Critical success index. *See* threat score

Cross-product ratio. *See* Diagnostic Odds
    Ratio (DOR)

D

Dementia, 1, 2, 5, 20, 21, 23, 25, 27, 28, 30,
    32, 34, 40, 42, 43, 46, 47, 49, 52,
    54, 55, 57, 58, 60–64, 66, 71–75,
    77, 79, 80, 82, 83, 85, 89, 90, 93,
    95, 96, 99, 100, 102–104, 107–109,
    113, 114, 116, 117, 119, 122, 125,
    126, 131, 135–137, 139, 141, 151,
    153–160, 162–165

Dementia CQUIN question, 19, 21

DemTect, 63, 64, 154, 160, 162

Depression, 2, 89, 99, 101, 103, 104

Diagnostic Odds Ratio (DOR), 3, 151

© Springer Nature Switzerland AG 2020
A. J. Larner, *Manual of Screeners for Dementia*,
https://doi.org/10.1007/978-3-030-41636-2